Neurostimulation

Principles and Practice

We dedicate this book to:

All healthcare professionals who decided to be involved in the care of patients who underwent neurostimulation.

Our teachers and mentors in functional neurosurgery, who enabled, empowered, and taught us the skills to implant neurostimulators and to take care of patients with neurostimulators.

Our students and fellows who made the jump onto functional neurosurgery to continue the art of functional neurosurgery in years to come.

All our patients for entrusting us to help them over the years via neurostimulation.

Our families for their support over the years, providing us with the best start in life, and education, and for their support during this project.

Professor Sam Eljamel
Professor Konstantin V. Slavin

Neurostimulation

Principles and Practice

Edited by

Sam Eljamel
Centre for Neurosciences
Ninewells Hospital & Medical School
Dundee, Scotland, UK

and

Konstantin V. Slavin
Department of Neurosurgery
University of Illinois at Chicago
Chicago, Illinois, USA

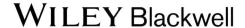

Registered office: John Wiley & Sons, Ltd, The Atrium, Southern Gate, Chichester, West
Sussex, PO19 8SQ, UK

Editorial offices: 9600 Garsington Road, Oxford, OX4 2DQ, UK
The Atrium, Southern Gate, Chichester, West Sussex, PO19 8SQ, UK
111 River Street, Hoboken, NJ 07030-5774, USA

For details of our global editorial offices, for customer services and for information about how
to apply for permission to reuse the copyright material in this book please see our website at
www.wiley.com/wiley-blackwell

Library of Congress Cataloging-in-Publication Data
Neurostimulation : principles and practice / edited by Sam Eljamel and Konstantin V. Slavin.
       p. ; cm.
   Includes bibliographical references and index.
   ISBN 978-1-118-34635-8 (hardback : alk. paper) – ISBN 978-1-118-34636-5 (ePub) –
ISBN 978-1-118-34637-2 (ePDF) – ISBN 978-1-118-34638-9 (eMobi) – ISBN 978-1-118-34639-6
(ebook online product)
   I. Eljamel, Sam.   II. Slavin, Konstantin V.
   [DNLM: 1. Central Nervous System Diseases–therapy.   2. Electric Stimulation Therapy.
3. Peripheral Nervous System Diseases–therapy.   4. Vagus Nerve Diseases–therapy. WL 300]
RM871
   615.8'45–dc23

                                                                         2013003017

A catalogue record for this book is available from the British Library.

Cover images: © 2013 St. Jude Medical, Inc. (main) and courtesy of Dr Alexander Green (inset)
Cover design by Andy Meaden

Set in 9/12.5 pt Interstate Light by Toppan Best-set Premedia Limited, Hong Kong
Printed and bound in Singapore by Markono Print Media Pte Ltd

1 2013

Contents

Colour plate section to appear between pages 84 and 85

List of Contributors

Editors

Sam Eljamel, MBBCh, MD, FRCS(Ed),(Ir),(SN)
Consultant Neurosurgeon, Centre for Neurosciences, University of Dundee,
Ninewells Hospital and Medical School, Dundee, UK

Konstantin V. Slavin, MD, FAANS
Head of Section of Stereotactic and Functional Neurosurgery, University of
Illinois at Chicago, Chicago, Illinois, USA

Contributors

Aviva Abosch, MD, PhD, FAANS
Neurosurgeon, Department of Neurosurgery, University of Minnesota,
Minneapolis, Minnesota, USA

Sami Al-Nafi, MD
Fellow in Functional Neurosurgery, Department of Neurosurgery,
University of Illinois at Chicago, Chicago, Illinois, USA

Giovanni Broggi, MD
Neurosurgeon, Fondazione Instituto Neurologico "Carlo Besta", Milan, Italy;
Department of Applied Neurosciences, Ludes University, Lugano,
Switzerland

Patrick Carena, BSC
Deputy Head of Instrumentation, Medical Physics, Ninewells Hospital and
Medical School, Dundee, UK

David Christmas, PhD
Consultant Psychiatrist, Advanced Interventions Service, Ninewells
Hospital and Medical School, Dundee, UK

Roberto Cordella, MD
Department of Neurosurgery, Fondazione Instituto Neurologico "Carlo
Besta", Milan, Italy

Pravin Dandegaonkar, MBBS, MD, FRCA, FCARCSI
Fellow in Pain Medicine and Specialty Registrar, Ninewells Hospital and
Medical school, Dundee, UK

Sam Eljamel, MBBCh, MD, FRCS(Ed),(Ir),(SN)
Consultant Neurosurgeon, Director of Functional Neurosurgery, University of Dundee, Ninewells Hospital and Medical School, Dundee, UK

Angelo Franzini, MD
Department of Neurosurgery, Fondazione Instituto Neurologico "Carlo Besta", Milan, Italy

Loes Gabriëls, PhD
Psychiatrist, KU Leuven, University Hospitals Leuven, Belgium

Gail Gillespie, MBChB, FRCA, FFPMRCA
Consultant in Anaesthesia and Pain Medicine, Regional Advisor in Pain Medicine for East of Scotland, Ninewells Hospital and Medical School, Dundee, UK

Eduardo Goellner, MD
Neurosurgeon, Hospital Mãe de Deus, Porto Alegre/RS, Brazil

Amit Goyal, MD
Fellow in Neurosurgery, University of Minnesota, Minneapolis, Minnesota, USA

Alexander Green, MD
Neurosurgeon, Department of Neurosurgery, John Radcliffe Hospital, Oxford, UK

Clement Hamani, MD
Neurosurgeon, Division of Neurosurgery, Toronto Western Hospital; University Health Network and Behavioural Neurobiology Laboratory, Centre for Addiction and Mental Health, Toronto, Ontario, Canada

Yasuaki Harasaki, MD
Fellow, Department of Neurosurgery, University of Colorado, Denver, Colorado, USA

Paul E. Holtzheimer, III, MD
Psychiatrist, Departments of Psychiatry and Surgery, Geisel School of Medicine at Dartmouth, Dartmouth Hitchcock Medical Center, Lebanon, New Hampshire, USA

Christopher R. Honey, MD, DPhil, FRCS(C)
Neurosurgeon, Department of Neurosurgery, University of British Columbia, Vancouver, British Columbia, Canada

Michael G. Kaplitt, MD, PhD, FAANS
Vice-Chairman for Research and Residency Director, Department of Neurological Surgery, Weill Cornell Medical College, New York, New York, USA

Antonios Mammis, MD
Resident, Department of Neurosurgery, University of Medicine and Dentistry of New Jersey, New Jersey Medical School, Newark, New Jersey, USA

Christine Matthews
Research Technician, Department of Psychiatry, University of Dundee, Dundee, UK

Keith Matthews, PhD
Psychiatrist, Division of Neuroscience (Psychiatry), Medical Research Institute, University of Dundee, Ninewells Hospital and Medical School, Dundee, UK

Giuseppe Messina, MD
Department of Neurosurgery, Fondazione Instituto Neurologico "Carlo Besta", Milan, Italy

Erwin B. Montgomery Jr., MD
Neurologist, University of Alabama, Birmingham, Alabama, USA

Ian Morrison, PhD, MRCP (UK)
Consultant Neurologist, Ninewells Hospital and Medical school, Dundee, UK

Steven Ojemann, MD, FAANS
Neurosurgeon, Department of Neurosurgery, University of Colorado, Denver, Colorado, USA

Manish Ranjan, MBBS, MCh
Fellow, Department of Neurosurgery, University of British Columbia, Vancouver, British Columbia, Canada

Serge Y. Rasskazoff, MD, FRCS(C)
Neurosurgeon, Flint, Michigan, USA

Michael Schulder, MD, FAANS
Professor and Vice Chairman, Department of Neurosurgery, Hofstra North Shore–LIJ School of Medicine, New York, New York, USA

Konstantin V. Slavin, MD, FAANS
Head of Section of Stereotactic and Functional Neurosurgery, University of Illinois at Chicago, Chicago, Illinois, USA

Serenella Tolomeo
Postgraduate Student, Department of Psychiatry, University of Dundee, Dundee, UK

Catherine Young, RCN
Specialist Movement Disorders Nurse, Ninewells Hospital and Medical School, Dundee, UK

Ludvic Zrinzo, MD, PhD, FRCSEd(NS)
Neurosurgeon, Sobell Department of Motor Neuroscience & Movement Disorders, UCL Institute of Neurology, University College London; Victor Horsley Department of Neurosurgery, National Hospital for Neurology and Neurosurgery, London, UK

Preface

Neurostimulation: Principles and Practice is intended to give a concise but comprehensive picture of the methods and devices which are now of use in neurostimulation to ameliorate the symptoms of Parkinson's disease (PD), tremor, dystonia, refractory epilepsy, chronic pain, depression and obsessive compulsive disorders. It should appeal to anyone training or working in the healthcare arena – whatever their particular discipline – who wants either a concise introduction to the subject, or a gentle reminder of stuff they might have forgotten. We have aimed the book at:

- Movement disorder neurologists, movement disorder specialist nurses, epileptologists, epilepsy specialist nurses, and residents in neurology.
- Pain specialists, pain specialist nurses and residents in pain management.
- Physicians of all grades who care for patients with PD, tremor, dystonia, chronic pain, or any patients who had a neurostimulator implanted.
- Psychiatrists and psychiatric specialist nurses with an interest in treatment refractory depression and OCD, and residents in psychiatry.
- Neurosurgeons interested in neurostimulation and neurosurgical residents.
- Any healthcare professional interested to learn more about neurostimulation.

This book is divided into sections on deep brain, motor cortex, vagus nerve, spinal cord, and peripheral nerve stimulation. Each section covers approved and emerging applications with chapters on each diagnosis and target to make it easier for healthcare professionals to navigate the text quickly to the desired information.

Neurostimulation: Principles and Practice is a systematic approach to understanding the mechanism of action, rationale, indications, patients' selection, targets, and programming of neurostimulators using common sense and the art of applying scientific knowledge to practice. No attempt is made to give detailed descriptions of surgical methods used to implant neurostimulators; these surgical methods have been adequately described in stereotactic books written specifically to neurosurgeons specializing in functional neurosurgery.

Contributors to this book were selected from around the globe because of their expertise and knowledge of each subject.

Professor Sam Eljamel
Centre for Neurosciences
Department of Neurosurgery
Ninewells Hospital & Medical School
Dundee, Scotland DD1 9SY, UK

Professor Konstantin V. Slavin
Department of Neurosurgery
University of Illinois at Chicago
912 S. Wood Street, M/C 799
Chicago, IL 60612, USA

Part 1
Deep Brain Stimulation

Chapter 1

Deep Brain Stimulation: Mechanisms of Action

Erwin B. Montgomery Jr.

University of Alabama, Birmingham, Alabama, USA

Introduction

Deep brain stimulation (DBS) is arguably the most effective treatment for movement disorders, such as Parkinson's disease (PD) and dystonia. DBS succeeds where all manner of pharmacological and biological therapies, such as neurotransplant, fail. Further, the range of disorders amenable to DBS is expanding rapidly, for example depression and epilepsy. At first, this may seem surprising, but that one would be surprised suggests a lack of appreciation that the brain is basically an electrochemical organ. The brain processes and transmits information electrically and, consequently, it should not be surprising that the brain's functions can be affected electrically. For example, while neurotransmitters, independently or affected by neuromodulators, result in changes in the electrical status in the post-synaptic neurons. The varying electrical changes induced by neurotransmitters are electrically integrated (processed) to produce new "information" that is subsequently encoded in the electric signal in the form of the axon potential train exiting the post-synaptic neuron. Further, changes in the neurotransmitter-induced post-synaptic electrical status produce further changes entirely independent of the neurotransmitter, such as post-excitatory depression of excitability due to deactivation of sodium (Na^+) conductance changes or post-inhibitory increases in excitability due to activation of Na^+ conductance channels among other voltage-sensitive conductance changes. Thus, for example, inhibition of the ventrolateral (VL) thalamus by activity in the globus pallidus interna (GPi), for many neurons results in a net increased VL neuronal activity contrary to what would be expected based on the neurotransmitter

Neurostimulation: Principles and Practice, First Edition. Edited by Sam Eljamel and Konstantin V. Slavin.
© 2013 John Wiley & Sons, Ltd. Published 2013 by John Wiley & Sons, Ltd.

released by GPi neurons onto VL neurons, that being gamma amino butyric acid (GABA) [1].

There has been a neurohumoral approach (analogous to an endocrine approach in terms of relative excesses or deficiencies in neurotransmitters or other chemical substances) to explain behavior since antiquity [2], and this was greatly reinforced with the discovery of neurotransmitters [3], the equating of neurotransmitter properties with electrical properties, and the rapid advances in pharmacology. Nevertheless, it would be an error of the category type (equating apples and oranges) derived from the fallacy of pseudo-transitivity (assuming similarity in one domain implies similarity in another domain) to equate neurotransmitter physiology to neurophysiology.

For example, the leading theories of basal ganglia pathophysiology and physiology focus on the GABAergic inhibition of the VL neurons. PD has been associated with overactivity of the GPi (falsely). The observation that destructive lesions of the GPi improved PD led to the false claim that similar benefits means that high-frequency DBS reduces activity in the GPi, via the fallacy of pseudo-transitivity. It is now clear that GPi DBS does not inhibit activity in GPi as measured by microelectrode recordings within the GPi or in VL thalamus [1,4]. Similarly, subthalamic nucleus (STN) DBS does not inhibit the output of the STN [5,6]. Recordings in VL thalamus do show a reduction in VL neuronal activity in the 3.5–7 ms following a GPi DBS pulse, but this is followed by a rebound in VL thalamic activity, such as through the thalamic neuron I_h channels and probably by reentrant feedback from the cortex [5]. For many VL neurons, GPi results in delayed increased neuronal activity, a phenomenon not accounted for in most theories of PD pathophysi-ology. Certainly, this effect on VL neurons could not have been predicted by what is known about GABA. Thus, the neuronal physiology is not synonymous with neurotransmitter function. It is my opinion that while the neurochemis-try and molecular biology of the basal ganglia have advanced rapidly, the understanding of the neurophysiology of the basal ganglia, more properly considered as the basal ganglia-thalamic-cortical system, has not. In large part this lack of progress in neurophysiology is that neurohumoral explana-tions have been thought sufficient.

Despite the remarkable advances in the clinical application of DBS since its first description in its modern form by Dieckmann for psychiatric disor-ders in 1979 [7] and by Cooper et al. for movement disorders in 1980 [8], little is known about the mechanisms of action of DBS. The lack of under-standing of the mechanisms of action is not for lack of studies. A PubMed search on "mechanism" and "DBS" results in 235 citations. To be sure, many have suggested a variety of possible mechanisms; however, most are incon-sistent with much of the experimental observations or do not or cannot provide a precise causal chain of events from injection of electrical charge into the brain with each DBS pulse to the behavior of motor units (the com-bination of a lower motor neuron and the muscle fibers it innervates).

This chapter begins with an attempt to answer the question as to what is the fundamental mechanism by which the DBS injection of electrical charge affects neurons. The implications of that answer for certain theories of DBS therapeutic mechanisms will be explored.

Importance of pathophysiological theories

Examination of the mechanisms of action of DBS did not and does not occur in a vacuum. Indeed, the popularization of DBS in the late 1980s and early 1990s despite the first use of DBS as it is done now in 1979 [7] and 1980 [8] is in large part due to the development of certain theories regarding the pathophysiology of movement disorders, particularly PD [9]. Indeed, the nature of theories of Parkinson pathophysiology current at the time directly shaped inferences as to DBS therapeutic mechanisms based on clinical effects. Later the prevailing theories of pathophysiology would shape what DBS experiments would have to be done, and what results were relevant and irrelevant as evidence. Indeed, it was the latter that was responsible for many errors in early DBS research resulting from confirmation bias.

The problem here is that it is very difficult to discuss DBS mechanisms without discussing the pathophysiological theories of the relevant neurological disorders that provides the context for DBS research. Indeed, these theories follow long antecedent conceptual approaches dating back to at least Aristotle. However, a full discussion is beyond the scope of this effort but this author's perspective has been published elsewhere [10,11,12,13,14]. Consequently, only specific aspects can be addressed here to provide some context to the issues related to DBS mechanisms.

The neuronal response to deep brain stimulation

This section surveys research observations regarding how individual neurons respond to the DBS pulse. A distinction is made between neuronal responses and neural responses. The former relates to individual neurons while the latter refers to the response of networks of neurons. This distinction is particularly important in view of the importance of DBS frequencies on therapeutic effects of DBS. As will be shown, the individual neuron's response to each DBS pulse is relatively the same despite DBS frequency, as shown in Figure 1.1 [5]. Consequently, the properties of the individual neurons are not likely to be the primary determinant of DBS because the frequency of DBS does have a specific effect on symptoms and the fact that the neuronal responses are the same means that the explanation of dependence on DBS frequencies for the therapeutic effect cannot be explained at the neuronal level. It is most likely that neural responses, that is the effects percolated throughout the basal ganglia-thalamic-cortical system are most relevant. Nevertheless, the neural network depends on driving activities within neurons; hence it is important to understand how neurons respond to DBS.

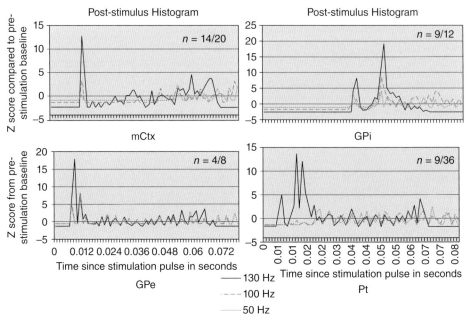

Figure 1.1 Post-stimulus histograms showing the changes in neuronal activity in the mCtx (motor cortex), globus pallidus interna (GPi), GPe (globus pallidus externa) and putamen (Pt) over the time interval from the onset of the subthalamic nucleus deep brain stimulation (DBS) pulse (time 0) to 8 ms after the DBS pulse (which is the interpulse interval for the 130 pps DBS). The ratio show the number of neurons demonstrating this pattern out of the total number of neurons recorded in that structure. The magnitudes of histograms have been z-score transformed and thus are in units of the value minus the mean of the pre-stimulation baseline divided by the standard deviation of the pre-stimulation baseline. As can be seen, the qualitative response in these neurons are relatively the same regardless of DBS frequency. However, there are quantitative differences in the magnitudes. The DBS frequencies typical of those clinically effective are associated with a greater magnitude of response. Reproduced from [13] with permission from Informa Healthcare.

As described earlier, the early theories of the therapeutic DBS mechanisms were inferred from the similarity of clinical efficacy of GPi and VL DBS to pallidotomy and thalamotomy, respectively. Thus, high-frequency DBS was thought to inhibit neuronal activity while low-frequency excites. As shown in Figure 1.1, this is not the case. However, as luck would have it, early neurophysiological studies appeared to provide support. Benazzouz et al. [15] recorded in the substantia nigra pars compacta while stimulating the STN in rodents and because they were unable to remove stimulus artifact, they studied the neuronal activity immediately following a DBS train of pulses. There was a reduction in neuronal activity, which was inferred to reflect activity during stimulation, which is now known to be a false inference. Recordings in the GPi with STN DBS demonstrate increased neuronal activity during stimulation with a profound reduction of GPi neuronal activity following cessation of DBS [5].

Most inferences of neuronal effects are related to direct microelectrode recordings. However, such recordings are highly selective of action potentials generated in the soma (cell body) and dendritic tree. Microelectrode recordings often demonstrated a reduction in extracellular action potentials in the stimulated target, with the inference that this was reflective of neuronal activity in general. This could reflect a tendency to think of a neuron primarily in terms of the soma and dendrites without appreciating the role of the axon. However, McIntyre and Grill [16] demonstrated, based on biophysical modeling, that action potentials could be generated in local axons despite reduced ability to generate action potentials in the soma and dendritic tree. Supportive neurophysiological observations in animals were rediscovered [17,18]. In addition to the biophysical explanation of reduced somatic and dendritic action potentials, it also was suggested that activation of pre-synaptic terminals, which have the lowest threshold to stimulation, resulted in somatic and dendritic hyperpolarization as the majority of pre-synaptic terminals are mediated by neurotransmitters that cause hyperpolarization in the post-synaptic neuron. Alternatively, some pre-synaptic neurotransmitters result in "shunting" inhibition in the soma and dendrites, rather than hyperpolarization, and have demonstrated reduction in action potentials in the soma and dendrites despite generation of action potentials in the axons [19].

Consequently, a therapeutic effect of DBS related to reduction in somatic and dendritic activity versus axonal output, for example in the STN, could not be distinguished. However, subsequent studies of therapeutic STN DBS demonstrated antidromic activation of the contralateral STN in patients whose ipsilateral PD symptoms were not worsened with STN DBS [20,21]. Consequently, STN overactivity is not a sufficient cause of PD nor is reducing STN neuronal activity a therapeutic mechanism of DBS (previous studies have shown that STN DBS activity is not greater than that recorded in the STN of patients with epilepsy and hence increased STN activity is not a necessary condition of PD [22]).

There is considerable evidence that DBS activates axons in the vicinity of the stimulating electrodes, whether they terminate in the stimulated target or are passing through the target. Evidence includes demonstrations of antidromic activation of cortical neurons with STN DBS [5,21] in response to STN DBS as well as in VL neurons in response to GPi DBS. Thus, it is entirely possible that the therapeutic effects of DBS may not have anything to do with activations of local neurons [23].

Another interesting phenomenon is that DBS is inefficient in activating neurons. For example, only on the order of 10-20% of DBS pulses result in an antidromic response [1]. The question is whether such inefficiencies are necessary for the DBS therapeutic effect. The hypothesis is that a certain degree of inefficiency is optimal for the DBS effect [12]. For example, some have argued that increasing DBS frequency or electrical current (voltage) results in a worsening effect on clinical symptoms. The precise mechanism is not clear; however, the explanation that spread to the internal capsule, at least in the case of STN DBS is not likely [12]. The hypothesis offered is that DBS resonates, and, hence, amplifies, neuronal activity within the basal ganglia-thalamic–cortical system in order to increase the signal-to-noise ratio to improve PD symptoms. In this case, the signal is the modulation of neuronal activity over time. However, there is a narrow range in which resonance would work. Insufficient activation of neurons will not amplify the signal. However, excessive driving of neurons will dampen the modulation by a ceiling effect.

DBS also synchronizes neuronal responses (Figure 1.1) as neurons have relatively stereotyped repetitive responses to the DBS pulses. Thus, DBS does not desynchronize neuronal activity within the basal ganglia-thalamic–cortical system as some have suggested. Further, recordings of motor unit activity (the summed muscle action potentials or muscle fibers simultaneously driven by an individual lower motor neuron) demonstrate synchronization with the DBS pulse [24]. Thus, if lower motor neurons are driven to synchronization with the DBS pulse, then it is very likely that the upper motor neuron in the motor cortex likewise is driven to synchronization with the DBS pulse. Whether or not this synchronization is due to antidromic activation of motor cortex neurons in the case of STN DBS [25] or by orthodromic activation accompanying antidromic activation of VL thalamic projection neurons is unknown.

The notion that DBS should desynchronize neuronal activities is derived by inverse inference that PD is consequent to abnormal synchronization of neuronal activities within the basal ganglia [26,27]. Further, computational simulations reinforced this notion. This suggests two caveats. First, inferring from the inverse is very problematic and may lead to false conclusions. Second, computational simulations often utilize powerful optimizing techniques. The consequence would be demonstration of plausible biological mechanisms that are not remotely true. Further, the misleading nature of computational simulations demonstrates the critical need for sufficient biological data to constrain the computational simulations.

To summarize the effects of DBS on neurons, the primary effect is depolarization of the neuronal membrane, which if the depolarization reaches threshold, an action potential is generated. Different neuronal elements have different thresholds. The lowest threshold is found in the pre-synaptic axonal terminals, the next lowest threshold is at the action potential initiating segment at the axon hillock or first inter-node, followed by the axon, and then finally by the soma and dendrites (some dendrites are capable of generating action potentials in terms of propagating regenerating changes in neuronal membrane potentials). Thus, perhaps the predominant effect is activation of pre-synaptic axonal terminals in the vicinity of the DBS electrodes and simultaneously, generation of action potentials of axons in the vicinity of the DBS electrodes. As many, if not most, pre-synaptic terminals release inhibitory neurotransmitters, the initial effect may be hyperpolarization of the somas and cell bodies in the vicinity of the DBS electrodes. This would be detected as a loss of action potentials recorded within the DBS target implying an inhibitory DBS effect. However, action potentials are generated in efferent axons such that the net effect is activation of the output of the stimulated structure. Recent evidence suggests that activation of the efferent axons is primary to the DBS effect and not the effect on the soma and dendrites of the DBS target. Generation of action potentials in the efferents of the DBS target then percolates throughout the network and it is this effect on the network that most likely is causal to the DBS therapeutic effect.

Neural responses to deep brain stimulation

The observations described earlier, call into question whether or not the direct neuronal responses to DBS are what mediate the therapeutic effects. The alternative is that it is the neural effects, meaning activations of the basal ganglia-thalamic-cortical system, that are required to effect the therapeutic response. Unfortunately, the vast majority of studies of DBS mechanisms have been confined to the stimulated target or structures monosynaptically downstream of the neurons within the stimulated target. The exception is a study in non-human primates with STN DBS-like stimulation, which demonstrates that the DBS-induced activity percolates through the entire basal ganglia-thalamic-cortical system (Figure 1.1). Further, these effects persist on the order of several milliseconds beyond the DBS pulse. Neither antidromic nor monosynaptic orthodromic mechanisms would explain the time course of the neuronal responses. Clearly, there is some additional means beyond direct driving by the DBS pulse that is determining the pattern of neuronal responses. A neural (polysynaptic) mechanism is most likely.

Further evidence of neural or network mechanisms underlying therapeutic DBS in the case of Parkinson's disease comes from evidence that DBS virtually anywhere within the basal ganglia-thalamic-cortical system is effective. For example, DBS of the GPi, GPe [28], VL, STN, motor cortex [29,30], and putamen [31] improve parkinsonian symptoms. Either there are as many therapeutic DBS mechanisms as there are targets or there is a single (or relatively few) and, consequently, the DBS is a system effect and not a structure effect. A system effect is more consistent with a neural response to DBS.

The systems oscillators theory posits that the basal ganglia-thalamic-cortical system can be conceived as a system of dynamically coupled re-entrant polysynaptic oscillators with non-linear properties (so as not to confuse with continuous harmonic oscillators), schematically represented in Figure 1.2 [13]. The system is made up of many oscillators of different lengths; hence, different inherent frequencies. The repetitive pulses of the DBS train interact via resonance, both positive and negative. Resonance of different oscillators within the basal ganglia-thalamic-cortical system with different DBS frequencies mediates the clinical responses to DBS of different frequencies [13].

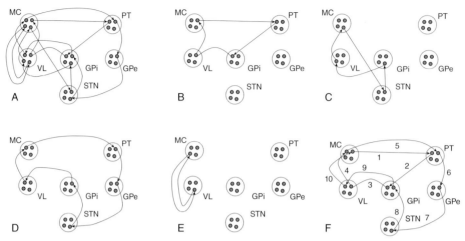

Figure 1.2 Schematic representations of the anatomical interconnections of some of the structures (A) within the basal ganglia–thalamic–cortical system where MC is the motor cortex, PT is putamen, GPe is globus pallidus externa, GPi is globus pallidus interna, STN is subthalamic nucleus, and VL is ventrolateral thalamus. Subsets of interconnections represent different possible oscillators (B-F) with different lengths represented by the number of nodes (collections of neurons) in the different structures. The different lengths result in different inherent or fundamental frequencies. Reproduced from [13] with permission from Informa Healthcare.

The concepts suggested by the Systems Oscillators theory are very different from current oscillator-based theories of PD pathophysiology, such as the beta oscillation theory [5,10,11,13,32]. This theory posits increased neuronal activity in the beta frequencies (8-30 Hz) as causal to PD. To be sure, increased power in the beta frequencies are seen in local field potentials recorded in various basal ganglia nuclei [33] which is reduced with levodopa administration or STN DBS. Similarly, DBS in the beta frequencies has been described as worsening PD symptoms, presumably by increased neural oscillations in the beta frequency. Consequently, DBS has been postulated to improve PD by reducing beta oscillations.

Figure 1.3 shows the hand opening and closing amplitudes and frequencies for a patient with STN DBS for PD at different DBS pulse rates [34]. As can be seen, there are multiple peaks in the amplitude and frequency, and DBS in the lower range of the beta frequencies improved motor performance. DBS in the higher beta frequencies did not worsen motor performance. Thus, the presence of beta oscillations, presumably resulting from DBS in the beta frequencies, is not a sufficient cause of PD, otherwise there would have been worsening of the PD symptoms.

Further, most studies of beta oscillations in local field potentials report composite or averaged data; in those few that show individual data there are some patients who do not display increased power in the beta oscillations. This demonstrates that increased beta power is not a necessary condition

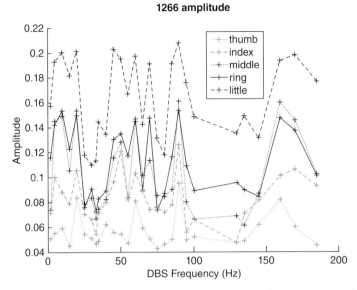

1266 amplitude

Figure 1.3 Mean relative amplitudes of the thumb and finger movements during a repetitive hand opening closing task. The mean amplitudes were from three trials at multiple subthalamic nucleus deep brain stimulation (DBS) frequencies. As can be seen, there are multiple distinct peaks over a wide range of frequencies, including in the beta range.

for PD because there are subjects who clearly have parkinsonism but do not have increased power in the beta frequencies. As beta oscillations is neither a necessary nor sufficient condition, it must be epiphenomena, in which case reduction in beta oscillations cannot be causal to PD, and thus, reduction of beta oscillations is not a therapeutic mechanism of action for DBS.

The results shown in Figure 1.3 suggest that improvements in hand opening-closing are improved at multiple but distinct frequencies. Second, the DBS stimulation rates that improve amplitude are not necessarily the same for hand opening-closing frequency suggesting different mechanisms, although what these mechanisms might be remains unknown. However, if DBS acts via resonance with ongoing oscillations within the basal ganglia-thalamic-cortical system, then the multiple peaks in improved motor performance suggests that there are multiple oscillators within the basal ganglia-thalamic-cortical system, as predicted by the systems oscillators theory, corresponding to the DBS frequencies associated with the peaks in the motor performance.

If the multiple peaks in motor performance associated with specific DBS rates are indicative of multiple and, consequently, independent oscillators within the basal ganglia-thalamic-cortical system, the question becomes what are the mechanisms that underlie these different oscillators and what are their specific roles in the function of the basal ganglia-thalamic-cortical system. At this point, one can only speculate and this is beyond the scope of this chapter, but there is a theory [13]. There is evidence that DBS does interact with oscillators within the basal ganglia-thalamic-cortical system. For example, as discussed above, STN DBS generates antidromic action potentials in the contralateral STN but only a fraction of the DBS pulses result in an antidromic action potential. Further study demonstrated that the antidromic action potentials were not random but periodic at 27 and 67 Hz, with many neurons showing both 27- and 67-Hz oscillations in the antidromic responses [35]. This suggests that the antidromic responses depend on the neuronal membrane potential and that the membrane potential oscillates at 27 and 67 Hz. As the 27 and 67 Hz are not commensurate (their ratio results in an irrational number), these oscillations must represent separate mechanisms. Further, the phase of the oscillations is different among STN neurons simultaneously recorded, suggesting that they represent different oscillators though at the same frequency.

It is likely that these oscillations at 27 and 67 Hz reflect polysynaptic reentrant neural oscillators, which are loosely coupled and non-linear. These mechanisms are feasible as demonstrated by mathematical simulations [36]. Assuming a conduction and synaptic delay between an action potential in one neuron and an increase in the membrane potential in the post-synaptic neuron (whether directly excitatory or post-inhibitory) of 3.7 ms, a 27-Hz oscillator suggests a 10-neuron (or node) oscillator within the basal ganglia-thalamic-cortical system. A 67-Hz oscillator suggests a four-neuron (or node) oscillator, such as motor cortex to putamen to GPi to VL back to motor cortex or a motor cortex to STN to GPi to VL and back to motor cortex.

Interestingly, STN DBS on the order of 67 Hz does not appear to improve motor performance (Figure 1.3), whereas DBS at twice that frequency appears optimal for motor performance. There are at least two possible explanations. First, it is possible that the STN DBS interacts with a two-neuron (or two-node) oscillator, such as the motor cortex-VL thalamus oscillator or the GPi–STN oscillator. Studies of VL neurons in response to GPi DBS may demonstrate such a phenomenon [5]. GPi DBS results in antidromic activation of VL neurons (Figure 1.4) [1]. This is followed by a reduction in VL neuronal activities consistent with activation of GPi axons projecting to the VL thalamus. This is followed by a slight rebound, though above pre-stimulation levels, which in turn is followed by a dramatic increase in activity at approximately 5 ms following the DBS pulse. However, there are subtle but telling changes in the antidromic and late activations. The late activations clearly can be seen to build, but at the same time there is a reduction in the antidromic response. There are at least two explanations. First, there is a build up of hyperpolarization in the VL neuron that blocks the antidromic activation, but this is not seen in the baseline activity that immediately follows where the antidromic response would have been. Alternatively, there may have been an action potential in the VL neuron (undetectable because it coincides with the stimulus artifact) that "collides" with the antidromic response, thereby preventing an action potential in the soma and dendritic tree of the VL neuron and, thus, no recordings of extracellular action potentials. This

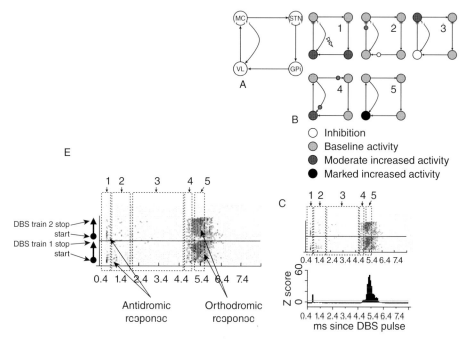

Figure 1.4 Example of post-stimulus rasters and histograms of the response of a ventrolateral (VL) neuron to globus pallidus interna (GPi) deep brain stimulation (DBS). E and C are rasters where each dot represents the discharge of a VL neuron during the inter-DBS pulse interval during high-frequency DBS. Note there are two separate trains of DBS (E). Each row represents the response to a single DBS pulse. The raster is "collapsed" by combining rows to produce the histogram seen in the bottom of C. As can be seen, there is a highly temporally consistent peak at approximately 0.8 ms following the DBS pulse consistent with antidromic activation (zone 1). There is a subsequent return of activity (zone 2) to baseline. At approximately 3.5 ms there is a reduction below baseline consistent with activation of GPi action potentials that then cause hyperpolarization of the VL neuron (zone 3). This is followed by a rebound increase in activity above baseline thought to represent post-inhibitory rebound excitability (zone 4). Later, there is a marked increase in neuronal activity (zone 5) thought to reflect feedback from activation of cortical neurons (most likely motor cortex (MC in A)). Evidence of a feedback mechanism is the progressive build up of the late response in zone 5; at the same time there is a reduction of the antidromic activity (zone 1). The most likely mechanism for reduction in the antidromic response is collision where an orthodromic action potential in the VL neuron, probably from the motor cortex, creates a refractory period that blocks an antidromic action potential from reaching the VL soma and dendrites where it could be recorded from the microelectrode in VL. This mechanism is schematically represented in A and B. A DBS pulse causes activation of the VL to motor cortex axon that results in an antidromic action potential being detected in the VL neuron (B1) and simultaneously, an orthodromic activation of the cortical neurons (B2 and B3). A few milliseconds later, the axonal activation of the GPi neuron results in release of GABA onto the VL neuron resulting in a reduction of activity (B2 and B3). At this time, the orthodromic activation of the motor cortex results in an action potential in motor cortex neurons (B3) that later results in orthodromic activation of the VL neurons (B5).

would explain why there is a progressive loss of antidromic responses as the late response builds, if one assumes that the late response is due to feedback from the motor cortex.

However, this would not explain the benefit of STN DBS at 250 Hz (not shown) in the hand opening–closing experiments described earlier, which would be too fast for any polysynaptic oscillator. Alternatively, supraharmonic DBS of a neural oscillator is effective for reasons that are unclear. One possible explanation is that the subsequent DBS pulse at 250 Hz falls on the post-refractory period increased excitability, for example due to activation of I_h channels or the greater activation of Na^+ channels induced by the prior pulse. Thus, a resonance amplification at the site of activation on the neuron could be related to the improvement of motor performance at 250-Hz DBS.

Higher order effects of deep brain stimulation

Whatever the therapeutic mechanisms of action of DBS for motor effects, it must correct the underlying abnormality in motor unit orchestration. The problem is that these abnormalities of motor unit control in movement disorders, such as PD, are poorly understood. Indeed, they are not understood because prior theories of basal ganglia pathophysiology never considered it necessary to explain motor unit control. Most theories posited that motor unit control was related to the biophysical properties of the lower motor neurons and thus, not affected by suprasegmental structures, such as the basal ganglia.

It is now clear that the abnormalities associated with motor unit control go far beyond simple one-dimensional push–pull dynamics of either general increases or decreases of motor unit activity. The Size Principle, which relates to the orderly recruitment of progressively larger motor units with increased force requirements, is abnormal and even reversed in some patients with PD [37]. In rapid movements, the relationships between the initial increase and then decrease in agonist electromyography, followed by an increase then decrease of antagonistic muscles, which in turn is followed by a final increase in the agonist muscle represents another higher level of motor unit orchestration that is abnormal in PD and current theories of PD pathophysiology, and therapeutic DBS mechanisms do not begin to explain these abnormalities.

The hypothesis offered here

Space limitations necessitate only a brief description of the alternative Systems Oscillators theory to explain basal ganglia pathophysiology and the therapeutic effects of DBS. Further explication and discussion of evidentiary support is offered elsewhere [5,10,11,13]. The basic premise is that the basal ganglia-thalamic cortical system is organized as numerous loosely coupled oscillators (Figure 1.2). The oscillators are constructed from reentrant connections between neurons. The nature of the interconnections is non-linear, which makes the oscillators discrete non-linear in contrast to typical harmonic continuous oscillators. The nodes of the oscillators comprise a subset of neurons within each of the nuclei and cortex of the basal ganglia-thalamic-cortical system. Thus, there may be many oscillators involved in given nuclei or cortex and the same neurons of a node may participate in multiple oscillators. Thus, an individual neuron may participate in multiple oscillators. Each neuron within a node does not discharge with each cycle of the oscillator but acts as a rate divider. Thus, the discharge activity of a neuron is less than the frequency of the oscillator in which it is embedded.

Because the oscillators are discrete, by virtue of the neurons in the node, they are discontinuous because of state changes that are different degrees of excitability and refractoriness. Similarly, thresholds from converting from continuous fluctuations in the membrane potential as inputs to discrete "all-or-nothing" action potentials at outputs mediated, conveys one aspect of non-linearity.

The discrete states and non-linear translations within the neurons confer unique properties on the basal ganglia-thalamic-cortical network, particularly related to interactions between oscillators. First, neurons of such systems are capable of simultaneously entraining multiple oscillators. Each oscillator serves as a carrier frequency to entrain information. The different frequencies of oscillations are related to a specific function that operates over a specific time scale. For example, the disynaptic VL motor cortex oscillator operates at high frequencies, approximately 147 Hz and, thus, can drive motor unit discharges at very short time scales. Conversely, the side-loops through the basal ganglia operate at lower frequencies to encode behaviors of a larger time scale, for example the temporal organization of agonist-antagonist-agonist muscle activations described earlier [13].

DBS acts as another oscillator within the basal ganglia-thalamic-cortical system. It acts as a loosely coupled oscillator because of the relative ineffectiveness of each DBS pulse to elicit an action potential [1]. Had the effectiveness been greater, the DBS would no longer act as a loosely coupled oscillator which would greatly change the dynamics within the basal ganglia-thalamic-cortical system [12]. In addition, the DBS oscillator is discrete because the DBS pulse, that is the time period by which it interacts with the other oscillators within the basal ganglia-thalamic-cortical system, is very brief relative to the interstimulus pulse interval.

The DBS oscillator then interacts with the basal ganglia-thalamic-cortical system depending on its frequency. For example, when the DBS oscillator is commensurate with specific basal ganglia-thalamic-cortical oscillators (which means that the ratio of their frequencies does not result in an irrational number), there can be interactions between these oscillators. However, if the DBS frequency is incommensurate with the frequency of a given oscillator the interaction becomes problematic or impossible.

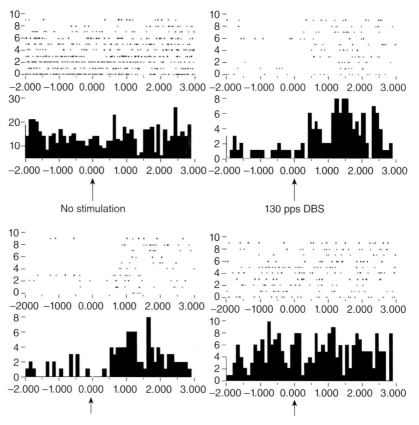

Figure 1.5 Peri-event rasters and histograms of a putamen neuron's activity in a non-human primate with a DBS-like system implanted in the subthalamic nucleus. The animal was trained to make an arm-reaching task in response to a go signal that occurred at time 0 and indicated by the upward arrow. The top of each figure shows rows of dots where each dot represents the discharge of the neuron. Each row represents the activities during a single trial of the task. The time scale is from 2 s before to 2 s after the go signal. The bottom parts of each figure are histograms from collapsing the rows above. As can be seen, under the no DBS condition, there is very little modulation of the neuronal activity relative to the go signal. At high frequency DBS, 130 pps, there is a remarkable modulation of the neuronal activity demonstrating the involvement of this neuron in task performance. At lower frequency DBS there is less modulation of neuronal activities. It is not likely that high-frequency DBS created the modulation of the neuronal activity as the DBS pulse train is constant. More likely, is that the modulation, representing a signal or information, was present but lost in the background activity. One possibility is that DBS at the proper frequency causes a resonance amplification of the underlying signal. Reproduced from [5] with permission from Elsevier.

The Systems Oscillators theory holds that the DBS pulse train can interact via positive and negative resonance to affect information encoded by the neuronal activities. Figure 1.5 demonstrates the effects of positive resonance on neuronal activity in the putamen. The converse, that is suppression of information also has been demonstrated and suggests that one action of DBS is to suppress misinformation [5].

The observations and hypotheses offered above present a novel conception of higher-level disorders in neurological and psychiatric disease. By higher level it is meant anything other than paralysis, in the case of movement disorders. This conception is that higher-level disorders are disorders of information causing misinformation rather than a loss or suppression of information. For example, the GPi rate theory posits that overactivity of the GPi in parkinsonism suppresses movement or blocks what would otherwise be normal information from reaching the motor cortex for subsequent expression.

Information implies a temporal dynamic, that is the modulation of neuronal and neural states over time. Further, the time scales over which information is encoded is on the order of milliseconds. For example, the difference in the structure of a therapeutic DBS at 150 pps and an ineffective DBS at 100 pps is an approximately 3.3 ms difference in the inter-DBS pulse intervals. Further, the relevant time scales are multiple and over a wide range as inferred from the multiple frequencies associated with the effects of STN DBS on hand opening–closing. It is highly unlikely that the one-dimensional push–pull dynamics that underlie much of the thinking about mechanisms of neurological and psychiatric disease and correspondingly about the mechanisms of DBS will provide anything close to a satisfactory explanation. Clearly, there must be an iterative process where explorations of DBS mechanisms cause changes in theories of pathophysiology, which in turn will affect the interpretations of DBS mechanisms. However, this will necessitate a revolutionary reassessment of modes of thinking going back to Aristotle [14]. At the very least, the therapeutic efficacy of DBS clearly re-establishes the primacy of the electrophysiological nature of brain function.

References

1 Montgomery, E.B., Jr (2006) Effects of GPi stimulation on human thalamic neuronal activity. *Clinical Neurophysiology*, **117**, 2691–2702.

2 Arikha, N. (2007) *Passions and Tempers: A History of the Humors*. HarperCollins Publisher, New York.

3 Valenstein, E.S. (2005) *The War of the Soups and Sparks: The Discovery of Neurotransmitters and the Dispute over How Nerves Communicate*. Columbia University Press, New York.

4 Anderson, M.E., Postupna, N. & Ruffo, M. (2003) Effects of high-frequency stimulation in the internal globus pallidus on the activity of thalamic neurons in the awake monkey. *Journal of Neurophysiology*, **89**, 1150–1160.

5 Montgomery, E.B., Jr & Gale, J.T. (2008) Mechanisms of action of Deep Brain Stimulation (DBS). *Neuroscience and Biobehavioral Reviews*, **32**, 388–407.

6 Reese, R., Gruber, D., Schoenecker, T. *et al.* (2011) Subthalamic deep brain stimulation increases pallidal firing rate and regularity. *Experimental Neurology*, **229**, 517-521.

7 Dieckmann, G. (1979) Chronic mediothalamic stimulation for control of phobias, *in* Modern Concepts. In: E.R. Hitchcock, H.T.J. Ballantyne & B.A. Meyerson (eds), *Modern Concepts in Psychiatric Surgery*, pp. 85-93. Elsevier, Amsterdam.

8 Cooper, I.S., Upton, A.R. & Amin, I. (1980) Reversibility of chronic neurologic deficits. Some effects of electrical stimulation of the thalamus and internal capsule in man. *Applied Neurophysiology*, **43**, 244-258.

9 Montgomery, E.B., Jr (2011) Commentary on neuromodulation perspectives. In: J.E. Arle & J.L. Shils (eds), *Essential Neuromodulation*, pp. 451-463. Elsevier, Amsterdam.

10 Montgomery, E.B., Jr (2004) Dynamically coupled, high-frequency reentrant, non-linear oscillators embedded in scale-free basal ganglia-thalamic-cortical networks mediating function and deep brain stimulation effects. *Nonlinear Studies*, **11**, 385-421.

11 Montgomery, E.B., Jr (2007) Basal ganglia physiology and pathophysiology: a reappraisal. *Parkinsonism and Related Disorders*, **13**, 455-465.

12 Montgomery, E.B., Jr (2010) *Deep Brain Stimulation Programming: Principles and Practice*. Oxford University Press, Oxford.

13 Montgomery, E.B., Jr & Gale, J.T. (2007) Neurophysiology and neurocircuity. In: R. Pahwa & K. Lyons (eds), *Handbook of Parkinson's Disease*, 4th ed., pp. 223-238. Informa Healthcare, New York and London.

14 Montgomery, E.B., Jr (2013) Neurophysiology. In: R. Pahwa & K. Lyons (eds), *Handbook of Parkinson's Disease*, 5th ed. Informa Healthcare, New York and London.

15 Benazzouz, A., Gao, D.M., Ni, Z.G. *et al.* (2000) Effect of high-frequency stimulation of the subthalamic nucleus on the neuronal activities of the substantia nigra pars reticulata and ventrolateral nucleus of the thalamus in the rat. *Neuroscience*, **2**, 289-295.

16 McIntyre, C.C. & Grill, W.M. (1999) Excitation of central nervous system neurons by nonuniform electric fields. *Biophysical Journal*, **76**, 878-888.

17 Llinas, R.R. & Terzuolo, C.A. (1964) Mechanisms of supraspinal actions upon spinal cord activities. Reticular inhibitory mechanisms on alpha-extensor motoneurons. *Journal of Neurophysiology*, **27**, 579-591.

18 Coombs, S.J., Curtis, D.R. & Eccles, J.C. (1957) The interpretation of spike potentials of motoneurons. *The Journal of Physiology (London)*, **39**, 198-231.

19 Dugladze, T., Schmitz, D., Whittington, M.A. *et al.* (2012) Segregation of axonal and somatic activity during fast network oscillations. *Science*, **336**, 1458-1461.

20 Novak, P., Klemp, J.A., Ridings, L.W. *et al.* (2009) Effect of deep brain stimulation of the subthalamic nucleus upon the contralateral subthalamic nucleus in Parkinson disease. *Neuroscience Letters*, **463**, 12-16.

21 Walker, H.C., Watts, R.L., Schrandt, C.J. *et al.* (2011) Activation of subthalamic neurons by contralateral subthalamic deep brain stimulation in Parkinson disease. *Journal of Neurophysiology*, **105**, 1112-1121.

22 Montgomery, E.B., Jr (2008) Subthalamic nucleus neuronal activity in Parkinson's disease and epilepsy patients. *Parkinsonism and Related Disorders*, **14**, 120-125.

23 Gradinaru, V., Thompson, K.R., Zhang, F. *et al.* (2009) Optical deconstruction of parkinsonian neural circuitry. *Science*, **324**, 354-359.

24 Aldewereld, Z.T. *et al.* (2012) *Effects of Deep Brain Stimulation on M-wave amplitude and motor unit cross-correlation in Parkinson's disease.* In *International Motoneuron Meeting*, 23-26 July 2012, Sydney Australia.

25 Walker, H.C., Huang, H., Gonzalez, C.L. *et al.* (2012) Short latency activation of cortex during clinically effective subthalamic deep brain stimulation for Parkinson's disease. *Movement Disorders*, **27**, 864-873.

26 Pogosyan, A., Yoshida, F., Chen, C.C. *et al.* (2010) Parkinsonian impairment correlates with spatially extensive subthalamic oscillatory synchronization. *Neuroscience*, **171**, 245-257.

27 Nini, A., Feingold, A., Nini, A. *et al.* (1995) Neurons in the globus pallidus do not show correlated activity in the normal monkey, but phase-locked oscillations appear in the MPTP model of parkinsonism. *Journal of Neurophysiology*, **74**, 1800-1805.

28 Vitek, J.L., Zhang, J., Hashimoto, T. *et al.* (2011) External pallidal stimulation improves parkinsonian motor signs and modulates neuronal activity throughout the basal ganglia thalamic network. *Experimental Neurology*, **233**, 581-586.

29 Benvenuti, E., Cecchi, F., Colombini, A. *et al.* (2006) Extradural motor cortex stimulation as a method to treat advanced Parkinson's disease: new perspectives in geriatric medicine. *Aging Clinical Experimental Research*, **18**, 347-348.

30 Drouot, X., Oshino, S., Jarraya, B. *et al.* (2004) Functional recovery in primate model of Parkinson's disease following motor cortex stimulation. *Neuron*, **44**, 769-778.

31 Montgomery, E.B., Jr, Huang, H., Walker, H.C. *et al.* (2011) High-frequency deep brain stimulation of the putamen improves bradykinesia in Parkinson's disease. *Movement Disorders*, **26**, 2232-2238.

32 Montgomery, J.E.B. (1994) A model of Parkinson's disease pathophysiology based on coupled oscillators. *Society for Neuroscience Abstracts*, **20**, 782.

33 Brown, P. (2006) Bad oscillations in Parkinson's disease. *Journal of Neural Transmission Supplementum*, **70**, 27-30.

34 Huang, H., Watts, R.L. & Montgomery, E.B.J. (2012) *Effects of DBS Frequencies on Hand Opening/Closing.* University of Alabama at Birmingham, Birmingham.

35 Montgomery, E.B., Jr, Huang, H., Guthrie, B.L. *et al.* (2012) Interactions of subthalamic nucleus antidromic action potentials and intrinsic oscillators. Program No. 380.17. *2012 Neuroscience Meeting Planner.* New Orleans, LA: Society for Neuroscience, 2012. Online.

36 Hoppensteadt, F.C. & Izhikevich, E.M. (1997) Weakly connected neural networks. In: J.E. Marsden, L. Sirovich & F. John (eds), *Applied Mathematical Sciences*, Vol. 126, pp. 275-285. Springer, New York.

37 Huang, H. *et al.* (2012) *Role of the basal ganglia in motor unit recruitment: effects of Parkinson's disease (PD) and Deep Brain Stimulation (DBS) of the subthalamic nucleus (STN).* In *International Motoneuron Meeting*. Sydney, Australia.

Chapter 2

Overview of Deep Brain Stimulation Components

Sam Eljamel

University of Dundee, Ninewells Hospital and Medical School, Dundee, UK

Deep brain stimulation components

Deep brain stimulation (DBS) consists of components surgically implanted by the surgeon and external components to communicate with the implanted device.

The implantable components consist of:

(1) **An implantable pulse generator (IPG)** houses the battery and electronic components that regulate the stimulation parameters. (Figure 2.1 gives some examples.)

    More than one company manufactures DBS systems and each IPG is able to drive current in a monopolar or bipolar fashion. The following parameters can be programmed: amplitude (Amp), pulse width (PW), rate (Hz), and active contacts. Table 2.1 compares some these IPGs currently in use.

(2) **An electrode implanted** into the brain target (DBS lead) (Figure 2.2). There are several DBS leads in the market (Table 2.2 gives a few examples) with a basic design consisting of four ring-type contacts labeled from distal to proximal.

(3) **Lead extender** that connects each lead to the IPG (Figure 2.3). Each DBS lead is compatible with a lead extender and each lead extender is compatible with an IPG (Table 2.3).

    The IPG is implanted in the left upper chest wall just below the collarbone (clavicle) or in the anterior abdominal wall using longer lead extenders. The junction between the DBS lead and the lead extender can be felt under the scalp often in the left parietal region.

(4) **Burr-hole caps** and DBS lead fixers: each vender of DBS system provides a burr hole cap to fix the DBS lead in place. The burr hole caps often felt as small hard swellings underneath the scalp incisions in the frontal scalp.

Neurostimulation: Principles and Practice, First Edition. Edited by Sam Eljamel and Konstantin V. Slavin.
© 2013 John Wiley & Sons, Ltd. Published 2013 by John Wiley & Sons, Ltd.

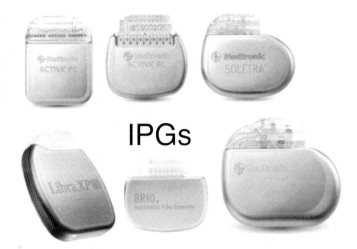

IPGs

Figure 2.1 Photograph of different implantable pulse generators for deep brain stimulation: Activa PC, RC, Soletra and Kinetra from Medtronic [1] (Soletra and Kinetra discontinued), LibraXP and Brio from St. Jude Medical [2]. Activa RC and Brio are rechargeable. Other venders are coming on the market, e.g., Boston Scientific [3]. Please check licenses for specific indications before using devices in patients.

Table 2.1 Comparison of implantable pulse generator models

IPG model	Kinetra	Activa RC	Activa PC	Activa SC	LibraXP	Brio
Thickness (mm)	15	9	15	11	14	10
Weight (g)	83	40	67	44	83	29
Header	Dual	Dual	Dual	Single	Dual	Dual
Amplitude	0-10.5 V	0-10.5 V	0-10.5 V	0-10.5 V	0-12.75 mA	0-12.75 mA
Pulse width (μs)	60-450	60-450	60-450	60-450	52-507	50-500
Rate Hz	3-250	10-250	2-250	2-250	2-200	2-240
No contact	0-7 (8)	0-7 (8)	0-7 (8)	0-3 (4)	1-8 (8)	1-8 (8)
PW steps (μs)	30	10	10	10	13	13
Amp steps	0.1 V	0.1 V	0.1 V	0.1 V	0.05 mA	0.05 mA
Volume (mL)	51	22	39	28	49	17.7

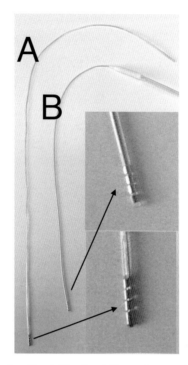

Figure 2.2 Deep brain stimulation lead dimensions and layout from two different venders: (A) St. Jude Medical; (B) Medtronic.

Table 2.2 Features of deep brain stimulation leads

Lead type	3387*	3389*	3391*	6143†	6147†
Length (cm)	40	40	40	40	40
Diameter (mm)	1.27	1.27	1.27	1.4	1.4
Contacts No.	0,1,2,3	0,1,2,3	0,1,2,3	1,2,3,4	1,2,3,4
Contact size (mm)	1.5	1.5	3	1.5	1.5
Contact space (mm)	1.5	0.5	4	1.5	0.5
Array length (mm)	10.5	7.5	24	12	9

*Medtronic.
†St. Jude Medical.

The non-implantable DBS components consist of:

(1) Physician Programmer

The Physician Programmer consists of a programming wand, a hand-held device that interrogates and transmits programming parameters between a DBS therapy computer and the IPG, and a hand-held or laptop computer that allows the physician to interrogate and programme the IPG (Figure 2.4).

(2) Patient's controllers

Patient's controllers are hand-held devices used by patients to switch the IPGs on/off and to increase or decrease the stimulation within a range of parameters set by the physician (Figure 2.5).

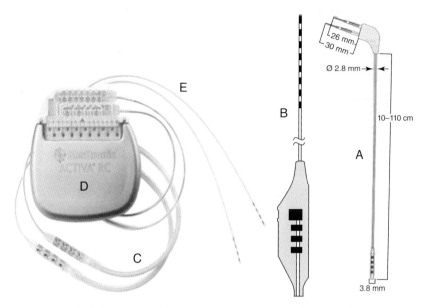

Figure 2.3 (A) Medtronic old lead extender; (B) St. Jude Medical lead extender; (C) new Medtronic lead extender attached to Activa RC (D) and deep brain stimulation leads (E).

Table 2.3 Lead extenders for deep brain stimulation leads

Lead extender	Medtronic 7483	Medtronic 37086	St. Jude Medical
Length (cm)	40-60-95	25-40-51-66-95	50-90
Thickness (mm)	2.7	1.3	1.4
Contacts	4	4	4
DBS end	3.8 mm	3.8 mm	5 × 7 mm
IPG end	Plug	Inline	Inline
Boot required	Yes	Yes	No

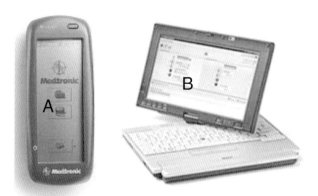

Figure 2.4 Photograph of the two most commonly used physician programmers in deep brain stimulation. (A) N'Vision from Medtronic; (B) Athena from St. Jude Medical.

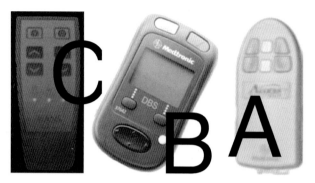

Figure 2.5 Patient's controllers: (A) Access for Kinetra; (B) Activa controller; (C) LibraXP controller.

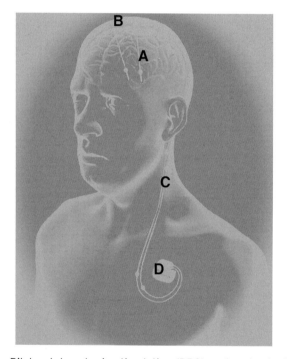

Figure 2.6 Bilateral deep brain stimulation (DBS) system implanted driven by one single dual channel IPG. (A) DBS lead; (B) the lead fixer/ burr hole cap; (C) lead extenders; (D) dual channel IPG. Reproduced with permission from St. Jude Medical.

(3) Chargers for rechargeable IPGs
   Some IPGs are rechargeable by patients, e.g., Activa RC from Medtronic and the Brio from St. Jude Medical.

Figure 2.6 depicts where the implanted components are located in most patients. However with longer lead extenders some patients prefer the IPG to be implanted in the abdominal wall. Stretchable lead extenders are also available giving much more flexibility particularly in dystonia.

References

1 Medtronic. Deep Brain Stimulation for Movement Disorders. http://professional.
medtronic.com/pt/neuro/dbs-md/prod/index.htm#tabs-1 [accessed on 6 March
2013].

2 St. Jude Medical. Leads and extension. http://www.sjmneuropro.com/Products/
Intl/DBS-Leads-and-extensions.aspx [6 March 2013].

3 Boston Scientific. Press Release. Boston Scientific Launches Vercise™ Deep
Brain Stimulation System in Europe http://phx.corporate-ir.net/phoenix.zhtml?
c=62272&p=irol-newsArticle&ID=1739324&highlight= [6 March 2013].

Chapter 3
Deep Brain Stimulation in Parkinson's Disease: Subthalamic Nucleus

Manish Ranjan and Christopher R. Honey

University of British Columbia, Vancouver, British Columbia, Canada

Introduction

The current popularity and widespread acceptance of deep brain stimulation (DBS) for Parkinson's disease (PD) began in the early 1990s after publications from teams in Grenoble [1,2] and Lille [3] introduced the concept of DBS to ameliorate abnormal movements without destroying tissue. DBS was appealing, because it was relatively safe, non-destructive, and its effects were reversible and could be titrated postoperatively. The most common targets for DBS in PD are the ventral intermediate nucleus (Vim) [4], globus pallidus internus (GPi) [5], and subthalamic nucleus (STN) [6]. Currently, DBS of the STN is the most common surgical procedure for PD. This chapter will highlight this operation and discuss (1) the rationale for neurostimulation of the STN, (2) referral criteria to select the ideal patient, (3) outcome, (4) stimulation parameters, and (5) potential side effects and complications.

Rationale for neurostimulation of subthalamic nucleus

The basal ganglia are a collection of four subcortical nuclei that modulate movement, composed of (1) the striatum, which includes the caudate and the putamen, (2) the external and internal segments of the globus pallidus (GPe and GPi), (3) the STN, and (4) the substantia nigra, which includes the pars compacta (SNc) and pars reticulata (SNr).

Neurostimulation: Principles and Practice, First Edition. Edited by Sam Eljamel and Konstantin V. Slavin.
© 2013 John Wiley & Sons, Ltd. Published 2013 by John Wiley & Sons, Ltd.

The striatum is the major input structure for the basal ganglia and receives excitatory glutamatergic projections from the cortex and dopaminergic projections from the SNc. Information is then relayed to the two output nuclei: GPi and SNr. The major outputs from the basal ganglia are inhibitory GABAergic (gamma aminobutyric acid) projections from the GPi and the SNr to the thalamus, which then projects to both the cortex and the pedunculopontine nucleus (PPN). The PPN projects back to striatum, basal ganglia, and cortex through ascending pathways and to the brain stem/spinal cord through descending pathways. The STN can also be considered an input nucleus because, like the striatum, it receives direct input from the cerebral cortex.

Within the basal ganglia there are two major pathways facilitating this neural network: the direct pathway and the indirect pathway. The direct pathway involves direct inhibitory GABAergic projections from the striatum to the output nuclei (GPi/SNr). Activation of this pathway inhibits the inhibitory output of the basal ganglia and results in increased activity of the excitatory thalamocortical projections. This direct pathway is thought to facilitate cortically initiated movement. The indirect pathway involves inhibitory projections from the striatum to the GPe. From the GPe there are inhibitory projections to the STN. The STN has excitatory glutamatergic projections to both output nuclei of the basal ganglia (GPi/SNr) and the GPe. Activation of the indirect pathway leads to increased inhibition of thalamocortical projections.

Normally, the dopaminergic output from the SNc facilitates activation along the direct pathway via excitatory D1 receptors in the striatum and inhibition along the indirect pathway via inhibitory D2 receptors. Dopaminergic output from the SNc therefore reduces the basal ganglia's inhibitory effect on thalamocortical neurons by both activating the direct pathway and inhibiting the indirect pathway. PD results in degeneration of the dopaminergic neurons within the SNc. The resultant loss of dopaminergic influence in the striatum results in increased activity in the basal ganglia output nuclei (GPi and SNr), and therefore pathological inhibition of the thalamocortical projections. Within the indirect pathway, the STN is pathologically activated (due to reduced inhibition from the GPe) and causes increased activity in both of the output nuclei of the basal ganglia. Destroying or modulating this pathologically increased activity in the STN of animal models of PD has been shown to ameliorate some of the symptoms of parkinsonism [7,8]. This model was the basis for suggesting that modulating the pathologic overactivity of the STN in PD patients would ameliorate their symptoms [6].

More recently, some researchers have questioned this simple model because it does not explain the genesis of symptoms such as tremor or dyskinesia. New models have been proposed incorporating information obtained during *in vivo* recordings in humans undergoing DBS (during microelectrode recording and local field potentials). These recordings revealed a rhythmic synchronized oscillatory local field potential within basal ganglia, with the most prominent activity being an increased synchronized oscillation in the beta band (13–30 Hz) of the pallidum and STN. Under normal information processing, there are complex spatiotemporal patterns of firing within STN and GPe. In PD, however, STN and GPe neurons display a correlated, synchronous, and rhythmic pattern of activity [9–13]. This pathological, synchronized, beta oscillatory activity is likely to result in less efficient coding of information within the basal ganglia and is linked to the symptoms of PD, especially bradykinesia. Furthermore, synchronous oscillatory activity in STN-GPe network is intimately related to rhythmic cortical activity, and since STN receives direct excitatory input from the primary motor cortex and supplementary motor area, it is likely that voluntary movements which modulate oscillatory phenomenon in the cortex might influence oscillatory synchronization in the STN. The STN is proposed to be important in the selection of wanted and the suppression of unwanted motor patterns and facilitates the desired motor movement. In one recent study of STN, local field potential during a go/no go task, beta activity in the STN correlated with slowness and was linked to the paucity of movement in PD [14]. These beta oscillations are suppressed by levodopa medication and DBS of the STN at high frequency. In contrast, stimulation of the STN at a beta frequency of 15 Hz worsened the parkinsonian disability through worsening of akinesia [15]. Synchronized beta oscillation in the STN is an electrophysiological hallmark of PD, and disrupting this synchronization may be how STN DBS exerts its beneficial effect.

In PD, another rhythmic bursting activity at 4–10 Hz has been observed and was phase locked with limb tremor in these patients [16,17]. Disruption of this rhythmic oscillatory electrical activity may be how STN DBS is able to reduce tremor in some PD patients [18].

PD is a diffuse synucleinopathy of the central nervous system with widespread neuronal involvement in olfactory, autonomic, limbic, and somatomotor systems. The early motor manifestations are likely due to the loss of dopaminergic cells in the SNc and consequent overactivity of STN with synchronized beta oscillation.

Referral criteria to select the ideal patient

Selecting the correct patient is equally important as performing the operation correctly. Both are required for a successful outcome.

Some excellent centers advocate STN DBS as the ideal target for all the cardinal symptoms of PD (tremor, rigidity, bradykinesia, and levodopa-induced dyskinesia). This is not our practice. We prefer Vim DBS for tremor-dominant PD, GPi DBS for disabling dyskinesia in otherwise mobile patients, lesions (pallidotomy and thalamotomy) for those who could not tolerate or choose not to have DBS, and reserve STN DBS for those with disabling "motor fluctuations." Motor fluctuations are transitions from an effectively medicated condition (often called the patient's "on" time or state) to an ineffectively medicated condition ("off"). Initially during the course of disease, symptoms typically respond very well to levodopa and the patient spends most of his/her time "on." With the progression of disease, however, the beneficial effect of a given dosage of levodopa tends to last for a shorter time and the patient begins to spend some of his/her time between doses in a less mobile "off" state. The specific symptoms during their "off" state will vary between patients but usually have some combination of rigidity, brady-kinesia, and tremor. Patients with advanced PD can sometimes fluctuate in their symptoms from bradykinetic-rigid to moving well (with or without peak dose dyskinesia) and then back to bradykinetic-rigid with each dose of their antiparkinsonian medication. These motor fluctuations can be modified ini-tially by adjusting the medications (shorting the dosage interval or adding enzyme inhibitors) but eventually they can become disabling in some patients. Determining when a symptom is disabling depends entirely on the individual patient. A similar magnitude of motor fluctuations may or may not be disa-bling depending on the patient's support system (family and care providers) and expectations.

STN DBS effectively reduces motor fluctuations and allows patients with advanced PD to spend more of their time "on" and less of their time "off." It has been observed that the preoperative response to levodopa is a good predictor of the postoperative response to STN DBS [19]. We therefore perform preoperative UPDRS (unified Parkinson's disease rating scale) testing in all surgical candidates. The UPDRS is made up of the following sections: part I: non-motor experiences of daily living (evaluation of mentation, behav-ior, and mood); part II: motor experiences of daily living (activities of daily life (ADLs)); part III: clinician-scored motor evaluation; and part IV: complica-tions of therapy [20]. The preoperative response to levodopa is measured by the percentage change in the UPDRS part III motor score measured "off" medications (following overnight withdrawal of PD medications) and "on" medications (following bolus of an ideal dose). Good surgical candidates will have at least a 30% improvement (reduction in score). We screen our surgi-cal candidates with the Montreal Cognitive Assessment (MoCA) to exclude those with dementia. Quality of life measures (SF 36 and Parkinson's disease questionnaire (PDQ) 39 [21]) are included to track our outcomes. Ideal can-didates have a clinically definitive diagnosis of idiopathic PD [22], have slowly progressive disease, have a good response to levodopa with their quality of life impaired by the symptoms that respond to levodopa, and have no cogni-tive impairment. They must have a clear understanding of what aspects of their PD will improve after surgery and they require a support system (family or friends) to ensure they get adequate follow-up care.

Contraindications

Contraindication to STN DBS can be both general and specific. General con-traindication to all DBS surgery include coagulopathy, uncontrolled hyper-tension, compromised healing or immune systems, inability for regular follow-up, and the expected need for future magnetic resonance scans near the implantable neural stimulator. Specific contraindications include symptoms not expected to improve following surgery such as freezing of gait in the "on" state or hypophonia. We do not consider advanced age as a surgical contraindication (some centers do not offer surgery to those >70 years). DBS can be considered in patients with cardiac pacemakers, provided both implanted devices are kept separate from each other and the manufacturer's guidelines are followed.

Outcome

STN DBS for PD was first reported by the Grenoble group [6]. They reported reversible restoration of movement without hemiballism or dyskinesia. STN DBS has subsequently been widely accepted for the treatment of patients with advanced PD. In 2001, the first prospective, double-blind study of DBS for PD (both STN and GPi) reported significant improvements in the UPDRS III motor score and increase in the "on" time [23]. Further, the effectiveness of STN DBS in both advanced and early-stage PD has been shown in prospective randomized controlled trials [24-26]. The beneficial result of STN DBS appears to be sustained with some studies following patients up to 10 years [27-29]. The clinical benefit of STN DBS was also found to be more effective than best medical management in a prospective randomized-pairs trial [25].

In a meta analysis of STN DBS, the average reduction in levodopa equivalents following surgery was 55.9% (95% CI: 50-61.8%), the average reduction in dyskinesia following surgery was 69.1% (95% CI: 62.0-76.2%), the average reduction in daily "off" periods was 68.2% (95% CI: 57.6-78.9%), and the average improvement in quality of life using PDQ 39 was 34.5% ± 15.3% [30]. STN DBS has clearly been established as an effective treatment for advanced PD.

Stimulation parameters

Initial device programming is typically delayed, as the surgical trauma usually causes a "microlesioning effect" and results in transient symptom improvement. The time course for this temporary microlesioning effect varies between patients. We typically begin our first programming 6 weeks postoperatively, once the patient has returned to their baseline preoperative status (some centers begin initial programming after 2 weeks). This avoids the confounding issue of a changing microlesion effect and the potential psychological stress of reduced clinical benefit after an initial excellent response to DBS.

STN DBS programming is typically based on the patient's rigidity, which responds within 20-30 s of stimulation. Bradykinesia and tremor also respond to STN DBS, but with a variable time gap. It is therefore ideal to have patients off their antiparkinsonian medicine prior to their first programming session.

Typically, the night dose of the medicine is withheld and the initial programming is done next morning to reduce patient discomfort. The patient's baseline neurological status should be documented and stimulation parameters (electrode polarity, contact, amplitude, pulse width, and frequency) chosen based upon the stimulation induced clinical benefits and adverse effects. Usually the electrode contact with the highest therapeutic window (i.e., benefit at low amplitude and adverse effect at high amplitude) in a monopolar setting is selected. The clinical benefit increases linearly with increasing frequency and is almost maximal around 130 Hz. There is a further small non-linear increase in efficacy above 130 Hz until a plateau is reached around 200 Hz [31]. Pulse width seems to have the least important role in improving clinical signs in the STN and is usually evaluated and set at 60 μs. The typical programming parameters for STN DBS are a monopolar setting using the contact with largest therapeutic window as cathode, pulse width of 60 μs, a frequency ≥130 Hz and the lowest amplitude (usual range 2–4 V) which provides clinical benefit with no adverse effects.

Potential side effects and complications

The STN is the most complex therapeutic target for DBS in PD in terms of surgery and programming owing to its very small size and the critical structures around it. Complications can be divided into surgical (perioperative), hardware (device related), and stimulation induced.

Surgical complications

Intracranial hemorrhage is the most dreaded complication. The incidence of hemorrhage in stereotactic and functional neurosurgery for movement disorders has been reported between 1.9% and 9.5% [23,32,33]. In a meta-analysis of reported complications following STN DBS, the incidence of hemorrhage was reported to be 3.9%. The proportion of patients who suffered a severe sequela was considerably lower [30]. Our impression has been that careful electrode trajectory planning with neuronavigation and judicious blood pressure management (<140 mmHg) during surgery are very helpful in avoiding such catastrophe. We have had no mortality and only two patients have developed symptomatic hemorrhage in more than 400 DBS cases.

Air embolism can occur during DBS surgery because the sitting position of the patient can place the surgical site (i.e., skull diploic space and dura) above the level of the heart. The incidence of air embolism in a large review of DBS cases was reported to be up to 3.2% [34]. This may be more relevant when working close to the midline (i.e., some approach trajectories for Vim DBS) but has been quite rare for STN DBS in our experience.

Transient confusion can follow STN DBS and has been reported as high as 15.6% [30]. This can be due to excessive cerebrospinal fluid (CSF) leakage with resulting pneumocephalus, brain shift, and trauma to the caudate nucleus from the electrode [30]. Preserving the arachnoid when opening the dura and then coagulating the arachnoid down onto the pia ("spot welding" the arachnoid to the pia) can reduce CSF leakage and reduce brain shift during surgery [35].

Hardware related

Problems related to the hardware include skin erosion (over the implantation site), infection, and malfunction of the device. There are reports of successful conservative management of skin erosion and infection [36,37], but frankly infected systems require explantation. The incidence of infection was reported to be 1.6% in a meta-analysis of STN DBS [30]. The same study reported reoperation to replace portions of the device in 4.4% of patients [30] due to malfunction, infection, or migration of the leads. We have reported that a curvilinear scalp incision (rather than straight incision) reduces the incidence of serious infection by keeping the hardware away from the incision [38].

Hardware breakage may result in a sudden loss of clinical benefit from DBS therapy. Testing the system's current and impedance may help identify this problem and an X-ray may localize the breakage.

Stimulation-related side effect

Stimulation of the STN can cause dyskinesia. Typically this is corrected by judicious reduction of the dopaminergic medication rather than reduction of stimulation. Stimulation-related side effects can also be due to unwanted spread of current and stimulation beyond the STN into adjacent neural pathways. These pathways include the corticospinal tract anterolaterally producing contralateral motor contraction, the medial lemniscus posteriorly causing contralateral paresthesia, the occulomotor nucleus and nerve medially causing ipsilateral eye deviation, and the frontal eye fields anteriorly causing forced contralateral gaze. These effects are transient and disappear when stimulation is reduced appropriately.

Occasionally some patients using monopolar settings complain of an abnormal sensation beneath the implantable pulse generator (IPG) (in the chest). "Buzzing" sensations at the IPG site can occur at high amplitudes and are completely stopped by switching the stimulation to a bipolar mode.

Some patients complain of a gradual loss of benefit from DBS therapy. This is a complex issue and might be attributable to inadequate stimulation, poor compliance of medicine, and/or progression of disease. Increasing the amplitude and frequency in conjunction with adjustment of medication may be helpful in some patients. The emergence of new, DBS-resistant symptoms (e.g., "on" freezing of gait) due to disease progression will not be effectively treated despite aggressive reprogramming.

Neuropsychiatric manifestations have been well described and can be quite dramatic in STN DBS [39,40]. Hypomania has been reported and is thought to be due to medial forebrain bundle fiber stimulation caudal to the STN [41]. There is an incidence of depression and suicide following STN DBS which may be multifactorial and needs further evaluation.

Conclusions

STN DBS is an effective add-on treatment for the carefully selected advanced PD patients with motor complications. It can improve quality of life by reducing "off" time and prolonging the patient's best "on" time. The patient's postoperative "on" time is typically no better than before surgery. Rather, they spend more time at that optimal "on" state following surgery. Like any operation, strict attention to surgical technique and close follow-up will reduce the incidence and impact of complications. It cannot be emphasized enough that excellent outcomes require both the selection of the correct patient and the operation to be performed correctly.

Further reading

Brown, P., Oliviero, A., Mazzone, P. et al. (2001) Dopamine dependency of oscillations between subthalamic nucleus and pallidum in Parkinson's disease. Journal of Neuroscience, **21**, 1033-1038.

Deep-Brain Stimulation for Parkinson's Disease Study Group (2001) Deep-brain stimulation of the subthalamic nucleus or the pars interna of the globus pallidus in Parkinson's disease. The New England Journal of Medicine, **345**, 956-963.

Dostrovsky, J. & Bergman, H. (2004) Oscillatory activity in the basal ganglia—relationship to normal physiology and pathophysiology. Brain: A Journal of Neurology, **127**, 721-722.

Honey, C.R. & Ranjan, M. (2012) Deep Brain Stimulation for Parkinson's disease—a review. European Neurological Review, **7** (1), 28-34.

Kleiner-Fisman, G., Herzog, J., Fisman, D.N. et al. (2006) Subthalamic nucleus deep brain stimulation: summary and meta-analysis of outcomes. Movement Disorders, **21** (Suppl. 14), S290-S304.

Moro, E., Esselink, R.J., Xie, J. et al. (2002) The impact on Parkinson's disease of electrical parameter settings in STN stimulation. Neurology, **59**, 706-713.

Moro, E., Lozano, A.M., Pollak, P. et al. (2010) Long-term results of a multicenter study on subthalamic and pallidal stimulation in Parkinson's disease. Movement Disorders, **25**, 578-586.

References

1 Benabid, A.L., Pollak, P., Louveau, A. et al. (1987) Combined (thalamotomy and stimulation) stereotactic surgery of the VIM thalamic nucleus for bilateral Parkinson disease. Applied Neurophysiology, **50**, 344-346.

2 Benabid, A.L., Benazzouz, A., Hoffmann, D. et al. (1998) Long-term electrical inhibition of deep brain targets in movement disorders. Movement Disorders, **13** (Suppl. 3), 119-125.

3 Blond, S. & Siegfried, J. (1991) *Thalamic stimulation for the treatment of tremor and other movement disorders. Acta Neurochirurgica Supplementum,* **52**, 109-111.

4 Benabid, A.L., Pollak, P., Seigneuret, E. *et al.* (1993) *Chronic VIM thalamic stimulation in Parkinson's disease, essential tremor and extra-pyramidal dyskinesias. Acta Neurochirurgica Supplementum,* **58**, 39-44.

5 Siegfried, J. & Lippitz, B. (1994) *Bilateral chronic electrostimulation of ventroposterolateral pallidum: a new therapeutic approach for alleviating all parkinsonian symptoms. Neurosurgery,* **35**, 1126-1129.

6 Benabid, A.L., Pollak, P., Gross, C. *et al.* (1994) *Acute and long-term effects of subthalamic nucleus stimulation in Parkinson's disease. Stereotactic and Functional Neurosurgery,* **62**, 76-84.

7 Aziz, T.Z., Peggs, D., Sambrook, M.A. & Crossman, A.R. (1991) *Lesion of the subthalamic nucleus for the alleviation of 1-methyl-4-phenyl-1,2,3,6-tetrahydropyridine (MPTP)-induced parkinsonism in the primate. Movement Disorders,* **6**, 288-292.

8 Bergman, H., Wichmann, T. & Delong, M.R. (1990) *Reversal of experimental parkinsonism by lesions of the subthalamic nucleus. Science,* **249**, 1436-1438.

9 Bergman, H., Wichmann, T., Karmon, B. & Delong, M.R. (1994) *The primate subthalamic nucleus. II. Neuronal activity in the MPTP model of parkinsonism. Journal of Neurophysiology,* **72**, 507-520.

10 Bergman, H., Feingold, A., Nini, A. *et al.* (1998) *Physiological aspects of information processing in the basal ganglia of normal and parkinsonian primates. Trends in Neurosciences,* **21**, 32-38.

11 Brown, P., Oliviero, A., Mazzone, P., Insola, A., Tonali, P. & Di Lazzaro, V. (2001) *Dopamine dependency of oscillations between subthalamic nucleus and pallidum in Parkinson's disease. Journal of Neuroscience,* **21**, 1033-1038.

12 Levy, R., Ashby, P., Hutchison, W.D., Lang, A.E., Lozano, A.M. & Dostrovsky, J.O. (2002) *Dependence of subthalamic nucleus oscillations on movement and dopamine in Parkinson's disease. Brain: A Journal of Neurology,* **125**, 1196-1209.

13 Wichmann, T. & Delong, M.R. (1996) *Functional and pathophysiological models of the basal ganglia. Current Opinion in Neurobiology,* **6**, 751-758.

14 Ray, N.J., Brittain, J.S., Holland, P. *et al.* (2011) *The role of the subthalamic nucleus in response inhibition: evidence from local field potential recordings in the human subthalamic nucleus. Neuroimage,* **60**, 271-278

15 Demeret, S., Bejjani, B.-P., Arnulf, I. *et al.* (1999) *Low frequency subthalamic stimulation worsens parkinsonian symptoms. Neurology,* **52** (Suppl. 2), A406.

16 Deuschl, G., Raethjen, J., Baron, R. *et al.* (2000) *The pathophysiology of parkinsonian tremor: a review. Journal of Neurology,* **247** (Suppl. 5), V33-V48.

17 Dostrovsky, J. & Bergman, H. (2004) *Oscillatory activity in the basal ganglia-relationship to normal physiology and pathophysiology. Brain: A Journal of Neurology,* **127**, 721-722.

18 Blahak, C., Bazner, H., Capelle, H.H. *et al.* (2009) *Rapid response of parkinsonian tremor to STN-DBS changes: direct modulation of oscillatory basal ganglia activity? Movement Disorders,* **24**, 1221-1225.

19 Charles, P.D., Van, B.N., Krack, P. *et al.* (2002) *Predictors of effective bilateral subthalamic nucleus stimulation for PD. Neurology,* **59**, 932-934.

20 Goetz, C.G., Tilley, B.C., Shaftman, S.R. *et al.* (2008) *Movement Disorder Society-sponsored revision of the Unified Parkinson's Disease Rating Scale (MDS-UPDRS): scale presentation and clinimetric testing results. Movement Disorders,* **23**, 2129-2170.

21 Jenkinson, C., Fitzpatrick, R., Peto, V., Greenhall, R. & Hyman, N. (1997) *The Parkinson's Disease Questionnaire (PDQ-39): development and validation of a Parkinson's disease summary index score. Age and Ageing*, **26**, 353–357.

22 Gelb, D.J., Oliver, E. & Gilman, S. (1999) *Diagnostic criteria for Parkinson disease. Archives of Neurology*, **56**, 33–39.

23 Deep-Brain Stimulation for Parkinson's Disease Study Group (2001) *Deep-brain stimulation of the subthalamic nucleus or the pars interna of the globus pallidus in Parkinson's disease. The New England Journal of Medicine*, **345**, 956–963.

24 Anderson, V.C., Burchiel, K.J., Hogarth, P. et al. (2005) *Pallidal vs subthalamic nucleus deep brain stimulation in Parkinson disease. Archives of Neurology*, **62**, 554–560.

25 Deuschl, G., Schade-Brittinger, C., Krack, P. et al. (2006) *A randomized trial of deep-brain stimulation for Parkinson's disease. The New England Journal of Medicine*, **355**, 896–908.

26 Schupbach, W.M., Maltete, D., Houeto, J.L. et al. (2007) *Neurosurgery at an earlier stage of Parkinson disease: a randomized, controlled trial. Neurology*, **68**, 267–271.

27 Castrioto, A., Meaney, C., Hamani, C. et al. (2011) *The dominant-STN phenomenon in bilateral STN DBS for Parkinson's disease. Neurobiology of Disease*, **41**, 131–137.

28 Moro, E., Lozano, A.M., Pollak, P. et al. (2010) *Long-term results of a multicenter study on subthalamic and pallidal stimulation in Parkinson's disease. Movement Disorders*, **25**, 578–586.

29 Rodriguez-Oroz, M.C., Obeso, J.A., Lang, A.E. et al. (2005) *Bilateral deep brain stimulation in Parkinson's disease: a multicentre study with 4 years follow-up. Brain: A Journal of Neurology*, **128**, 2240–2249.

30 Kleiner-Fisman, G., Herzog, J., Fisman, D.N. et al. (2006) *Subthalamic nucleus deep brain stimulation: summary and meta-analysis of outcomes. Movement Disorders*, **21** (Suppl. 14), S290–S304.

31 Moro, E., Esselink, R.J., Xie, J., Hommel, M., Benabid, A.L. & Pollak, P. (2002) *The impact on Parkinson's disease of electrical parameter settings in STN stimulation. Neurology*, **59**, 706–713.

32 Terao, T., Takahashi, H., Yokochi, F. et al. (2003) *Hemorrhagic complication of stereotactic surgery in patients with movement disorders. Journal of Neurosurgery*, **98**, 1241–1246.

33 Binder, D.K., Rau, G.M. & Starr, P.A. (2005) *Risk factors for hemorrhage during microelectrode-guided deep brain stimulator implantation for movement disorders. Neurosurgery*, **56**, 722–732.

34 Hooper, A.K., Okun, M.S., Foote, K.D. et al. (2009) *Venous air embolism in deep brain stimulation. Stereotactic and Functional Neurosurgery*, **87**, 25–30.

35 Coenen, V.A., bdel-Rahman, A., McMaster, J. et al. (2011) *Minimizing brain shift during functional neurosurgical procedures - a simple burr hole technique that can decrease CSF loss and intracranial air. Central European Neurosurgery Journal*, **72**, 181–185.

36 Lanotte, M., Verna, G., Panciani, P.P. et al. (2009) *Management of skin erosion following deep brain stimulation. Neurosurgical Review*, **32**, 111–114.

37 Fenoy, A.J. & Simpson, R.K., Jr (2012) *Management of device-related wound complications in deep brain stimulation surgery. Journal of Neurosurgery*, **116**, 1324–1332.

38 Constantoyannis, C., Berk, C., Honey, C.R. *et al.* (2005) *Reducing hardware-related complications of deep brain stimulation. The Canadian Journal of Neurological Sciences*, **32**, 194-200.

39 Hariz, M.I. (2002) *Complications of deep brain stimulation surgery. Movement Disorders*, **17** (Suppl. 3), S162-S166.

40 Hariz, M.I., Rehncrona, S., Quinn, N.P. *et al.* (2008) *Multicenter study on deep brain stimulation in Parkinson's disease: an independent assessment of reported adverse events at 4 years. Movement Disorders*, **23**, 416-421.

41 Coenen, V.A., Honey, C.R., Hurwitz, T. *et al.* (2009) *Medial forebrain bundle stimulation as a pathophysiological mechanism for hypomania in subthalamic nucleus deep brain stimulation for Parkinson's disease. Neurosurgery*, **64**, 1106-1114.

Chapter 4

Deep Brain Stimulation in Parkinson's Disease: Pallidal (globus pallidus pars interna)

Yasuaki Harasaki and Steven Ojemann
University of Colorado, Denver, Colorado, USA

Introduction

The first reports of stereotactic lesioning procedures specifically targeting the globus pallidus pars interna (GPi) for idiopathic Parkinson's disease (PD) occurred in 1953. Guiot and Brion [1] described electrocoagulation of the anterodorsal GPi, while Narabayashi et al. [2]. independently reported chemical lesioning of the same target. It was noted that while there was lasting improvement in rigidity, the effect on hypokinesia and tremor were not lasting.

Lars Leksell began pallidotomies with the same target in 1952, but, dissatisfied with the results, began to explore alternative targets. A prospective study of 81 patients undergoing lesioning of various targets was published in 1960 by Svennilson et al. [3]. The best results were obtained from the last patients of the series, who had undergone posteroventral pallidotomies. Of the 20 patients in this group, 19 derived lasting benefit from the procedure [3].

Surgical lesioning procedures largely went out of favor with the introduction of levodopa and dopamine agonist therapy in the late 1960s. With the observation that these treatments lost effectiveness in many patients over time, and that chronic use of levodopa was associated with debilitating dyskinesias, interest was again kindled in the possibility of pallidotomies for patients who failed or were unable to tolerate medical therapy.

In 1992, Laitinen et al. [4] published clinical results on a series of 38 patients who had undergone posteroventral pallidotomies with significant improvements in hypokinesia, tremor, and rigidity, as well as improvement

Neurostimulation: Principles and Practice, First Edition. Edited by Sam Eljamel and Konstantin V. Slavin.
© 2013 John Wiley & Sons, Ltd. Published 2013 by John Wiley & Sons, Ltd.

or resolution in levodopa-induced dyskinesias. Subsequently, with the increasing popularity of deep brain stimulation (DBS) since the 1990s, the GPi has remained a target of interest in idiopathic PD.

Rationale of globus pallidus pars interna deep brain stimulation in Parkinson's disease

The choice of target for DBS has been a topic of ongoing debate. To date, the best-studied targets have been the subthalamic nucleus (STN) and the GPi. A study by the Deep Brain Stimulation for Parkinson's Disease Study Group in 2001 showed significant improvement in motor function, with stimulation of either the STN or the GPi, an effect which on follow-up study was shown to be durable at 24 months [5,6]. However, there was significant reduction in the dose of levodopa required by the patients at 6 months with stimulation of the STN but not of GPi. Based on this finding, which has been replicated in additional studies [7,8], the STN has become the target of choice for stimulation in idiopathic PD at many centers.

Recently, however, it has been proposed that the STN has an inhibitory role not only in movement disorders but also in behavior. Impulse control disorders have been well-known complications of dopamine agonist therapy [9]. It has also been noted that DBS of the STN in particular appears to have higher risk of behavioral side effects, particularly with impulsivity [10]. Frank and coworkers [10] proposed a computational model in which the STN provides a "hold your horses" signal in response to high-conflict decisions. During the more difficult high-conflict decision tasks, normal controls and patients with STN DBS turned off had appropriately longer response latencies than low-conflict tasks. The same patients with activated STN stimulation tended to respond more quickly and make more errors in the high-conflict tasks [10]. A second, more recent model proposes that the role of the STN is one of "proactive inhibition," in which it provides a more general tonic inhibitory signal in executive control to suppress inappropriate automatic responses to irrelevant stimuli [11].

The effects of DBS on cognition and mood are also currently under investigation. A recent large-scale Veterans Affairs Cooperative study showed some decrement in neurocognitive function in all patients undergoing DBS, but showed a more pronounced decrement in processing speed index (Wechsler Adult Intelligence Scales III) in the STN group at 24-month follow-up. Over the same period, there was an improvement in the GPi group and slight worsening in the STN group of the Beck Depression Inventory II. Both STN and GPi groups experienced similar improvements in motor function and quality of life [5].

GPi stimulation also appears to be more effective in directly inhibiting dyskinesia than STN stimulation, which relies on reduction in dopamine agonists for its antidyskinetic effect [12]. At 3 months post initiation of GPi stimulation, a 65-75% reduction in dyskinesia scores was noted. This effect appears to be durable, with a persistent 50% reduction in dyskinesia scores evident at 3 years postoperatively [12].

There have been recent calls for re-evaluation of the GPI over the STN as preferred target [13], but at this time, the possibility of reduction in dopaminergic agents favors the STN as the primary target in DBS for PD. GPi DBS may be an option for the subset of patients with dyskinesia as a predominant symptom, more atrophy on imaging studies, marginal preoperative neuropsychological findings, or pre-existing psychiatric or behavioral comorbidity.

Patient selection and referral criteria

General patient selection criteria for DBS in PD are similar for both the STN and the GPi and will be briefly reviewed here (Table 4.1). While one study showed that shortly following Food and Drug Administration approval of DBS, only 4.5% of referred patients were appropriate candidates for DBS [14], more recent data suggest that referral patterns have significantly improved in the intervening years [15].

For patients who are being referred to GPi rather than STN DBS due to a question of cognitive or psychiatric risk, preoperative referral for neurocognitive and/or psychiatric testing including the Beck Depression Inventory II remains critical.

Targeting

Surgical placement of electrodes in the GPi is most commonly performed using a direct targeting strategy, as the lateral coordinates of the GPi varies considerably between individuals. Excellent visualization of the pallidal structures, and importantly the pallidocapsular border on magnetic resonance imaging (MRI) can be achieved with various imaging sequences [16,17].

Table 4.1 Traditional patient criteria for deep brain stimulation for Parkinson's disease [15]

Clear diagnosis of idiopathic Parkinson's disease

Disabling motor fluctuations despite adequate medical therapy, and/or disabling levodopa-induced dyskinesias

Lack of significant cognitive impairment

Lack of significant medical comorbidities

Lack of untreated psychiatric comorbidities

Lack of structural abnormality or significant atrophy of the brain on magnetic resonance imaging

Realistic expectations of outcomes and possible complications

Adequate social support, ability to participate in postoperative follow-up

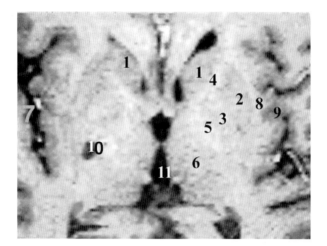

Figure 4.1 Axial volumetric MRI demonstrating the caudate head (1), anterior limb (4) and posterior limb (5) of the internal capsule, the thalamus (6), the putamen (2), the GPi (3) and a pallidotomy lesion in the right GPi (10), (7) the insula, (8) external capsule and (9) Insular cortex.

Targeting is performed in our center using the method described by Starr [18]. A plane containing the intercommissural (anterior commissure-posterior commissure) line is chosen, and the pallidocapsular border is identified in this plane. Next, the length of the pallidum along the pallidocapsular border is measured; generally this is around 18 mm. A target through which the trajectory will pass is defined by measuring anteromedial one-third the length of the pallidum (i.e., 6 mm for an 18-mm pallidocapsular length) and then 3-4 mm anterolateral from this point along a line perpendicular to the pallidocapsular line. The point at the end of this line should fall approximately 1 mm from the GPi–GPe lamina (Figure 4.1).

This will define a point through which the trajectory will pass. The entry point is defined on the surface along a trajectory that is approximately 60 degrees relative to the intercommissural line in the sagittal plane, and the trajectory is as close as possible to the parasagittal plane, as long as this does not traverse the ventricle or a deep sulcus. With the entry point defined, the trajectory is extended approximately 4 mm beyond the targeted point in the intercommissural plane, such that it will typically terminate at the superolateral edge of the optic tract.

Intraoperative microelectrode recording can be used to confirm electrode position. The electrode first traverses the GPe prior to entering the GPi. Two types of cells are encountered in the GPe. One exhibits tonic low-frequency discharge of around 20 Hz with irregular high-frequency bursts of 300-500 Hz. Another fires at 40-60 Hz with intermittent pauses. The GPi, in contrast, has higher frequency discharges of 70-120 Hz with fewer pauses [19].

A silent tract with tonic muscle contraction indicates an electrode in the internal capsule, placing it too medial or posterior to the optimal tract.

Patient report of phosphenes or increased firing rate noted with light stimulation in the eyes signifies the placement of the electrode in the optic tract, making it too ventral [19,20].

Programming parameters

Stimulation is generally initiated with the patient in the medication-off state. As with stimulation of the STN, the initial programming parameters for GPi stimulation is amplitude 0.1, pulse width 60 or 90 μs, and frequency of 130–160 Hz [21]. The amplitude is incrementally increased for all electrode combinations to optimize the therapeutic effect while minimizing adverse effects. Some clinicians prefer sequential monopolar stimulation with each electrode to rapidly determine the optimal locus of stimulation.

Differential effects of stimulation of the ventral and dorsal GPi have been described. External GPi is thought to induce dyskinesia, while internal GPi improves dyskinesia but worsens bradykinesia [20]. The goal of electrode selection is to stimulate the transition zone between these functional zones in the lateral posteroventral GPi.

Complications of globus pallidus pars interna deep brain stimulation

DBS remains a safe procedure. Binder and coworkers [22] examined hemorrhage associated with DBS in a series of 481 lead implantations and found overall risk of 3.3%. There was a significant difference in hemorrhage by target, with 7.0% for GPi, 2.2% for STN, and 1.2% for thalamus ($p = 0.001$).

The Veterans Affairs Cooperative Studies Program examined 299 patients with bilateral lead implantation in either STN ($n = 147$) or GPi ($n = 152$). At 2-year follow-up, 50.7% of patients in the GPi group and 56.5% in the STN group had experienced serious adverse events leading to death, disability, or prolonged or new hospitalization. The three most common adverse events were implantation site infection, fall, and pneumonia. Hemorrhage rates were 2.7% for GPi versus 1.4% for STN. There were no significant differences in adverse events by type between the STN and GPi groups [5].

References

1 Guiot, G. & Brion, S. (1953) Treatment of abnormal movement by pallidal coagulation. *Revue Neurologique*, **89** (6), 578–580.
2 Narabayashi, H., Okuma, T. & Shikiba S. (1956) Procaine oil blocking of the globus pallidus. *A. M. A. Archives of Neurology and Psychiatry*, **75** (1), 36–48.
3 Svennilson, E., Torvik, A., Lowe, R. & Leksell, L. (1960) Treatment of parkinsonism by stereotatic thermolesions in the pallidal region. A clinical evaluation of 81 cases. *Acta Psychiatrica Scandinavica*, **35**, 358–377.

4 Latitinen, L.V., Bergenheim, A.T. & Hariz, M.I. (1992) Leksell's posteroventral pallidotomy in the treatment of Parkinson's disease. *Journal of Neurosurgery*, **76**, 53–61.

5 Follett, K.A., Weaver, F.M., Stern, M. *et al.* (2010) Pallidal versus subthalamic deep-brain stimulation for Parkinson's disease. *The New England Journal of Medicine*, **362** (22), 2077–2091.

6 Deep-Brain Stimulation for Parkinson's Disease Study Group (2001) Deep-brain stimulation of the subthalamic nucleus or the pars interna of the globus pallidus in Parkinson's disease. *The New England Journal of Medicine*, **345** (13), 956–963.

7 Rodriguez-Oroz, M.C., Obeso, J.A., Lang, A.E. *et al.* (2005) Bilateral deep brain stimulation in Parkinson's disease: a multicentre study with 4 years follow-up. *Brain: A Journal of Neurology*, **128** (Pt 10), 2240–2249.

8 Anderson, V.C., Burchiel, K.J., Hogarth, P. *et al.* (2005) Pallidal vs subthalamic nucleus deep brain stimulation in Parkinson disease. *Archives of Neurology*, **62** (4), 554–560.

9 Weintraub, D., Koester, J., Potenza, M.N. *et al.* (2010) Impulse control disorders in Parkinson disease: a cross-sectional study of 3090 patients. *Archives of Neurology*, **67** (5), 589–595.

10 Frank, M.J., Samanta, J., Moustafa, A.A. *et al.* (2007) Hold your horses: impulsivity, deep brain stimulation, and medication in parkinsonism. *Science*, **318** (5854), 1309–1312.

11 Ballanger, B., van Eimeren, T., Moro, E. *et al.* (2009) Stimulation of the subthalamic nucleus and impulsivity: release your horses. *Annals of Neurology*, **66** (6), 817–824.

12 Toda, H., Hamani, C. & Lozano, A. (2004) Deep brain stimulation in the treatment of dyskinesia and dystonia. *Neurosurgical Focus*, **17** (1), E2.

13 Tagliati, M. (2012) Turning tables: should GPi become the preferred DBS target for Parkinson disease? *Neurology*, **79** (1), 19–20.

14 Okun, M.S., Fernandez, H.H., Pedraza, O. *et al.* (2004) Development and initial validation of a screening tool for Parkinson disease surgical candidates. *Neurology*, **63** (1), 161–163.

15 Katz, M., Kilbane, C., Rosengard, J. *et al.* (2011) Referring patients for deep brain stimulation: an improving practice. *Archives of Neurology*, **68** (8), 1027–1032.

16 Reich, C.A., Hudgins, P.A., Sheppard, S.K. *et al.* (2000) A high-resolution fast spin-echo inversion-recovery sequence for preoperative localization of the internal globus pallidus. *AJNR. American Journal of Neuroradiology*, **21** (5), 928–931.

17 Sudhyadhom, A., Haq, I.U., Foote, K.D. *et al.* (2009) A high resolution and high contrast MRI for differentiation of subcortical structures for DBS targeting: the Fast Gray Matter Acquisition T1 Inversion Recovery (FGATIR). *Neuroimage*, **47** (Suppl. 2), T44–T52.

18 Starr, P.A., Turner, R.S., Rau, G. *et al.* (2004) Microelectrode-guided implantation of deep brain stimulators into the globus pallidus internus for dystonia: techniques, electrode locations, and outcomes. *Neurosurgical Focus*, **17** (1), E4.

19 Danish, SF, Moyer, JT, Jaggi, JL. (2007) Neurophysiology of the microelectrode track during subthalamic nucleus and globus pallidus internus targeting. In: G.H. Baltuch & M.B. Stern (eds), *Deep Brain Stimulation for Parkinson's Disease (Neurological Disease and Therapy)*, pp. 99–100. Informa Healthcare, New York.

20 Yelnik, J., Damier, P., Bejjani, B.P. et al. (2000) Functional mapping of the human globus pallidus: contrasting effect of stimulation in the internal and external pallidum in Parkinson's disease. *Neuroscience*, **101**, 77–87.
21 Johnson, L. & Kumar, R (2010) Managing Parkinson' s disease patients treated with deep brain stimulation. In: W.J. Marks (ed.), *Deep Brain Stimulation Management*, pp. 62–82. Cambridge University Press, Cambridge.
22 Binder, D.K., Rau, G.M. & Starr, P.A. (2005) Risk factors for hemorrhage during microelectrode-guided deep brain stimulator implantation for movement disorders. *Neurosurgery*, **56** (4), 722–732.

Chapter 5

Deep Brain Stimulation of the Pedunculopontine Nucleus for Parkinson's Disease

Aviva Abosch and Amit Goyal

University of Minnesota, Minneapolis, Minnesota, USA

Introduction and background

Parkinson's disease (PD) is the second most common neurodegenerative disorder, affecting almost 1% of the population over the age of 60 years and nearly 4% of the population over the age of 80 years [1]. It is a major cause of morbidity and mortality in elderly people and accounts for well over $20 billion in annual healthcare expenses in the USA alone. Typically manifesting in the fifth or sixth decade of life, PD has four cardinal features: resting tremor, bradykinesia, rigidity, and postural instability. Although resting tremor in the hand is the first symptom noticed in almost three-quarters of PD patients [2], postural and gait instability may in fact be the most worrisome. Injuries from falls substantially increase the morbidity associated with the disease and account for the vast majority of visits to the Emergency Department for this patient population.

DBS has become the most widely used surgical intervention for the treatment of PD. The two main targets of DBS for PD are the subthalamic nucleus (STN) (Chapter 3) and globus pallidus pars interna (GPi) (Chapter 4), both of which have shown similar efficacy in alleviating parkinsonian motor symptoms [3]. Although the benefit of STN and GPi stimulation on motor fluctuations, tremor, bradykinesia, rigidity, and dyskinesia is now well documented, Visser and colleagues [4] demonstrated that neither GPi nor STN stimulation improves levodopa-resistant postural instability. Because of the severe impact that postural instability and gait disturbance have on patients' lives, there has been increased interest in identifying alternate targets for DBS, in

Neurostimulation: Principles and Practice, First Edition. Edited by Sam Eljamel and Konstantin V. Slavin.
© 2013 John Wiley & Sons, Ltd. Published 2013 by John Wiley & Sons, Ltd.

an effort to treat these symptoms. The most promising target under investigation is the pedunculopontine nucleus (PPN).

Characterization of the pedunculopontine nucleus

The PPN is located in the rostral locomotor region of the pons and midbrain and has been implicated in wide-ranging studies in the control of posture and in the initiation and maintenance of gait [5]. Located medial to the medial lemniscus, lateral to the decussation of the superior cerebellar peduncle, caudal to the substantia nigra, and rostral to the cuneiform nuclei (Figure 5.1), the PPN does not possess a true nuclear structure but is instead defined by its two major groups of neurons—the *pars compacta* (PPNc), and the *pars*

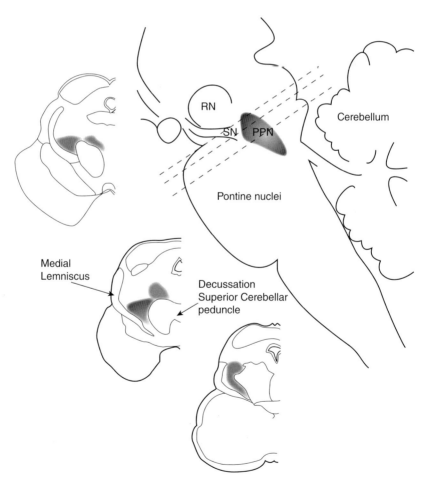

Figure 5.1 Anatomical location of the PPN. RN, red nucleus; PPN, pedunculopontine nucleus; SN, substantia nigra. Reproduced from [6] with permission from Wiley.

dissipatus (PPNd). PPNc contains densely packed cholinergic neurons, whereas PPNd is characterized by glutaminergic output [6].

The PPN is densely interconnected with the basal ganglia and thalamus, but its exact role in modulating pallidothalamic output is not fully understood. The PPN receives major input from the GPi and substantia nigra reticulata, as well as moderate input from the STN. PPN neurons project to nearly all the basal ganglia nuclei, but most densely to the SNc and STN. The PPN also has ascending cholinergic and glutaminergic projections to the thalamus. In addition to its afferent and efferent connections with the basal ganglia and thalamus, the PPN has ascending and descending connections to numerous other structures throughout the central nervous system, including the motor cortex and spinal cord [6].

Rationale for targeting the pedunculopontine nucleus

The PPN arose as a site of interest in the pathophysiology of PD in the 1980s. In post-mortem studies of PD patients, researchers observed the hallmark degeneration of dopaminergic neurons located in the substantia nigra compacta (SNc). Yet, they also noted as much as a 50% loss of cholinergic neurons in the PPN and suggested that this degeneration might also be associated with the disease process [7]. With this information, researchers began focusing studies on the function and role of the PPN, exploring its potential as a surgical target in the treatment of PD.

Since then, a variety of studies have continued to support the PPN as a promising target. Animal studies, following on the heels of the postmortem findings in PD patients, demonstrated that PPN stimulation induced locomotion in decerebrate rats. In addition, lesioning of this area caused akinesia in otherwise normal primates [8]. Both findings further supported the importance of PPN in initiation and maintenance of gait.

An important leap occurred in 2002 when Nandi and colleagues [9] linked the PPN to PD in animal models. Lesioning of the PPN in a normal-behaving primate caused akinesia whereas injection of the GABA antagonist bicuculline into the PPN alleviated akinesia in a monkey treated with the PD-inducing drug, 1-methyl-4-phenyl-1,2,3,6-tetrahydropyridine (MPTP). This provided a proof-of-concept that the PPN could serve as a focal point for correcting posture and gait in patients with PD. When Jenkenson *et al.* [10] demonstrated in 2004 that stimulation of the PPN improved akinesia in monkeys treated with MPTP, they reinforced the relevance of the PPN in PD-related gait disturbance and proposed the PPN as a novel DBS target for the treatment of PD. The link between the PPN and gait was further underscored when Kuo *et al.* [11] published in 2008 that bilateral PPN strokes produced significant gait freezing.

The animal studies performed over the last two and a half decades have led to the suggestion that disinhibition of PPN in patients with PD might alleviate freezing episodes and prevent falls. As a consequence, over the past

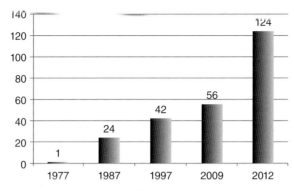

Figure 5.2   Number of pedunculopontine nucleus stimulation citations by year.

several years, the number of studies devoted to PPN stimulation has increased exponentially as researchers have strived to establish PPN as a viable option in the treatment of PD (Figure 5.2).

Results from recent clinical studies of pedunculopontine nucleus stimulation

As investigations of the PPN as a therapeutic target have moved into clinical studies, results have continued to suggest that the site provides a means to address postural instability and gait dysfunction. In small groups of patients, initial studies of PPN DBS reported significant improvements in the debilitating axial symptoms associated with PD [12,13]. Subsequent clinical investigations have attempted to document the safety and efficacy of PPN stimulation in patients with PD (Table 5.1). Despite promising results, however, PPN stimulation remains investigational in North America and Europe.

In the first clinical study, published in 2007, Stefani *et al.* [14] incorporated PPN stimulation into the treatment of six patients with PD. The subjects presented with primary symptoms of severe postural instability and impairment of gait, despite optimal medical management. All six patients underwent bilateral PPN *and* STN DBS lead placement for the treatment of disabling symptoms. Results from this open-label study demonstrated that low-frequency bilateral PPN stimulation alone (25 Hz, 60 s, 2 V, bipolar configuration) did not offer an improvement in *overall* unified Parkinson's disease rating scale (UPDRS) motor scores compared with bilateral STN stimulation alone. However, when combined with bilateral STN stimulation, the addition of PPN stimulation *did* provide a significant benefit for several important axial symptoms. Specifically, when patients were in the "on" medication state and underwent PPN stimulation, they were noted to more easily rise from a seated position, had improved posture, displayed better gait, and had improved postural stability via the pull test (items 27–30 of the motor UPDRS

Table 5.1 Summary of recent studies of PPN stimulation for Parkinson's disease

Author (year)	Number of patients	Target(s)	Primary outcome measures	Results	Study design
Stefani et al. (2007)	6	Bilateral PPN + bilateral STN	N/A	Significant improvement in UPDRS scores on items 27-30 for STN + PPN stimulation	Open-label; no randomization
Moro et al. (2010)	6	Unilateral PPN	Total scores of the UPDRS parts II and III and the sub-scores of UPDRS items 13, 14, 29, and 30	Subjective, self-reported symptom improvement; no objective improvement in overall group UPDRS scores	Double-blind; no randomization
Ferraye et al. (2010)	6	Bilateral PPN + Bilateral STN	Composite gait score, Giladi questionnaire, and data from the walking protocol	Subjective, self-reported symptom improvement; no objective improvement in overall group UPDRS scores	Double-blind crossover study during months 4–6
Thevathasan et al. (2011)	5	Bilateral PPN	Gait and Falls Questionnaire	Subjective, self-reported symptom improvement; no objective improvement in overall group UPDRS scores	Open-label; no randomization

STN, subthalamic nucleus; PPN, pedunculopontine nucleus.

scores). These observed benefits were documented immediately after lead placement and noted to be sustained at 6 months [14].

In another study, published in 2010, Moro et al. [15] investigated the effects of unilateral PPN stimulation. The study examined six PD patients whose postural abnormalities were causing substantial compromise in quality of life due to freezing of gait and/or falls, symptoms believed to be resistant to

STN stimulation. The results of this double-blind investigation demonstrated that PPN stimulation (50-70 Hz, 60 s, 2 V, bipolar configuration) produced a significant improvement in *self-reported* falls (68%) and freezing of gait (67%) at 3 and 12 months, even though *overall* objective UPDRS scores remained unchanged.

Ferraye *et al.* [16] reported the results of the first prospective, double-blinded, crossover investigation of bilateral PPN stimulation in six PD patients in 2010. Each of the patients suffered predominantly from gait freezing and instability contributing to falls. All of the patients had previously undergone DBS with lead placement in the STN; all six had additional leads placed in the PPN for this study. During the first 3 months after surgery, patients underwent stimulation of both sites with known settings. During months 4-6, researchers conducted the double-blind crossover study with low-frequency PPN stimulation (15-25 Hz, 60 s, 1.2-3.8 V, bipolar configuration) versus sham stimulation. For the sham stimulation, researchers went through the motions of initiating stimulation without actually activating the device. Researchers then tracked the number of falls, episodes of freezing, gait, and postural stability. The results of the study were similar to those reported by Moro and colleagues: although researchers found no *objective* improvement in motor UPDRS scores for the entire group, patients reported significant improvement. At 24 months after surgery, patients reported fewer freezing episodes and related falls. These researchers recommended that further randomized studies be conducted to determine the efficacy of PPN stimulation.

In 2011, Thevathasan *et al.* [17] studied bilateral stimulation of the PPN in an open-label investigation. The five patients in the study had severe symptoms of gait freezing, postural instability, and falls. These patients had not been considered candidates for STN stimulation because despite being optimized on medical therapy, their primary symptoms remained those of gait and postural instability. With low-frequency bilateral PPN stimulation, patients reported significant improvement in self-assessment of freezing, balance disturbance, and falls on the Gait and Falls Questionnaire, which was administered at 6 months and 2 years following onset of stimulation. As in previous studies, the PPN did not improve UPDRS scores on items 27-30 for the group as a whole, nor did it reduce dopaminergic medication requirements [17]. For two of the patients tested at 2 years of follow-up, however, scores for items 27-30 did show improvement under specific circumstances. Although patients demonstrated better scores when in the on-medication, on-stimulation state (compared with off-stimulation scores), neither researchers nor patients were blinded to the stimulation conditions.

Limitations of current studies

The results of the studies to date suggest that PPN stimulation is safe and that it holds promise for the treatment of postural instability and freezing of gait associated with PD. However, limitations in the design of these published studies obligate further investigation prior to a definitive statement regarding efficacy. Future studies would benefit from larger sample size, longer postoperative follow-up, randomization between treatment and control arms, and blinding of raters and study subjects to therapy condition (stimulation versus sham). In addition, studies will have to take into consideration the limitations of the experimental setting because gait freezing and falls are far more common at home than in the clinic environment [18]. Also of benefit would be the inclusion of formal gait and postural testing, such as computerized dynamic posturography, in order to provide objective and quantitative analysis of patient gait and posture.

A criticism that has been raised regarding some of the publications mentioned pertains to the specificity of PPN targeting. The human PPN is difficult to identify with microelectrode recordings or MRI [19] because it lacks distinct borders. It has been described as a reticular structure, belonging to the mesencephalic reticular formation. Yelnik [20] disputed the location of electrode implantation in the study by Stefani et al. [14], suggesting that, according to the Schaltenbrand and Wahren Atlas [21], researchers implanted electrodes in the peripeduncular nucleus (PPD), and not the PPN. Zrinzo and colleagues [19], while studying methods on how best to identify the PPN, noted a significant difference in localization of the rostral and caudal poles of the PPN depending on whether researchers used atlas-based coordinates or relied upon direct visualization with MRI. Because of these inconsistencies, authors are increasingly using the term pedunculopontine nucleus *area* (PPNa) to describe the target region [16].

Further analysis will doubtless verify the precise location for PPN electrode implantation in patients undergoing DBS surgery. Improving PPN imaging protocols will ensure accurate placement of electrodes in the PPN. With better imaging and electrophysiologically based localization, it will be possible to eliminate variation in electrode placement between patients and standardize the outcome of stimulation.

Potential complications and adverse effects

The complications associated with DBS surgery, which primarily include intracranial hemorrhage and hardware-related infection, have been well documented elsewhere. Adverse effects specifically related to stimulation of the PPN include oscillopsia (see later) [15,17,22]. Paresthesia may occur [14,15], most likely due to the close proximity of the PPN to the medial lemniscus. Patients may also experience transient changes in pain and temperature sensation [15,16], believed to be caused by excitation of the spinothalamic tract [14,16]. Myoclonus, which has also been reported following low-frequency stimulation of the ventral intermediate nucleus of the thalamus, is believed to be a consequence of stimulation of PPN fibers projecting to the thalamus [16].

Ferraye et al. [22] reported "trembling vision" in 33% of patients ($n = 2$) who underwent PPN stimulation, suggesting interference with the oculomotor fibers of the mesencephalic region from stimulation. Although abnormal eye movements were not observed clinically, oculomotor recordings revealed frequency-locked, voltage-dependent vertical or oblique movements of the eye ipsilateral to the active DBS contact. Jenkinson and colleagues [23] have argued instead that stimulation of the fibers of the uncinate fasciculus of the cerebellum and superior cerebellar peduncle causes stimulation of the saccadic premotor neurons of the brainstem, resulting in PPN stimulation-induced oscillopsia. Thevathasan et al. [17] reported oscillopsia at higher voltage settings in all of their patients ($n = 5$), but found that it was easily prevented with slower voltage escalation (over the course of hours to weeks). Moro et al. [15] reported oscillopsia in 83% of patients ($n = 5$) and an abnormal sensation of warmth in 50% of patients ($n = 3$).

Although transient, paresthesia occurred in all patients who underwent PPN stimulation, according to both Stefani et al. [14] ($n = 6$) and Moro et al. ($n = 6$) [15]. Myoclonus (both positive and negative) of the limbs was reported by Stefani et al. [14] in 33% of patients ($n = 2$). Ferraye et al. [16] noted that myoclonus occurred in all of their patients ($n = 6$), but that the symptom was also easily and completely reversed by simply decreasing the voltage of stimulation.

Conclusions

Although STN and GPi stimulation provides significant benefit for PD-related motor fluctuations and tremor not responsive to medication, interest continues to grow in investigating the efficacy of PPN stimulation as therapy for postural instability and gait disturbances associated with the disease. Although recent studies suggest that PPN stimulation is safe and may provide benefit for axial symptoms, this therapy remains investigational. Sustained efficacy, using objective and quantitative measures of gait performance, has yet to be established in large groups of patients. Future investigations should address the exact location of PPN in order to standardize and optimize electrode placement. While preliminary results have been encouraging, longer-term, randomized controlled studies with larger patient populations and standardized objective clinical assessment are needed to definitively establish the efficacy of PPN stimulation. The addition of PPN as a target for DBS provides a promising approach to treat the potentially dangerous axial symptoms of postural instability and gait disturbance that plague PD patients.

References

1 de Lau, L.M.L. & Breteler, M.M.B. (2006) Epidemiology of Parkinson's disease. *Lancet Neurology*, **5**, 525-535.

2 Jankovic, J. (2008) Parkinson's disease: clinical features and diagnosis. *Journal of Neurology, Neurosurgery, and Psychiatry*, **79**, 368-376.

3 Follett, K.A., Weaver, F.M., Stern, M. *et al.* (2010) Pallidal versus subthalamic deep-brain stimulation for Parkinson's disease. *The New England Journal of Medicine*, **362**, 2077-2091.

4 Visser, J.E., Allum, J.H., Carpenter, M.G. *et al.* (2008) Subthalamic nucleus stimulation and levodopa-resistant postural instability in Parkinson's disease. *Journal of Neurology*, **255**, 205-210.

5 Aziz, T.Z., Davies, L., Stein, J. & France, S. (1998) The role of descending basal ganglia connections to the brain stem in parkinsonian akinesia. *British Journal of Neurosurgery*, **12**, 245-249.

6 Jenkinson, N., Nandi, D., Muthusamy, K. *et al.* (2009) Anatomy, physiology, and pathophysiology of the pedunculopontine nucleus. *Movement Disorders*, **24**, 319-328.

7 Hirsch, E.C., Graybiel, A.M., Duyckaerts, C. *et al.* (1987) Neuronal loss in the pedunculopontine tegmental nucleus in Parkinson disease and in progressive supranuclear palsy. *Proceedings of the National Academy of Sciences of the United States of America*, **84**, 5976-5980.

8 Garcia-Rill, E., Houser, C.R., Skinner, R.D. *et al.* (1987) Locomotion-inducing sites in the vicinity of the pedunculopontine nucleus. *Brain Research Bulletin*, **18**, 731-738.

9 Nandi, D., Aziz, T.Z., Liu, X. *et al.* (2002) Brainstem motor loops in the control of movement. *Movement Disorders*, **17**, S22-S27.

10 Jenkinson, N., Nandi, D., Miall, R.C. *et al.* (2004) Pedunculopontine nucleus stimulation improves akinesia in a parkinsonian monkey. *Neuroreport*, **15**, 2621-2624.

11 Kuo, S.H., Kenney, C. & Jankovic, J. (2008) Bilateral pedunculopontine nuclei strokes presenting as freezing of gait. *Movement Disorders*, **23**, 616-619.

12 Mazzone, P., Lozano, A., Stanzione, P. *et al.* (2005) Implantation of human pedunculopontine nucleus: a safe and clinically relevant target in Parkinson's disease. *Neuroreport*, **16**, 1877-1881.

13 Plaha, P. & Gill, S.S. (2005) Bilateral deep brain stimulation of the pedunculopontine nucleus for Parkinson's disease. *Neuroreport*, **16**, 1883-1887.

14 Stefani, A., Lozano, A.M., Peppe, A. *et al.* (2007) Bilateral deep brain stimulation of the pedunculopontine and subthalamic nuclei in severe Parkinson's disease. *Brain: A Journal of Neurology*, **130**, 1596-1607.

15 Moro, E., Hamani, C., Poon, Y.Y. *et al.* (2010) Unilateral pedunculopontine stimulation improves falls in Parkinson's disease. *Brain: A Journal of Neurology*, **133**, 215-224.

16 Ferraye, M.U., Debu, B., Fraix, V. *et al.* (2010) Effects of pedunculopontine nucleus area stimulation on gait disorders in Parkinson's disease. *Brain: A Journal of Neurology*, **133**, 205-214.

17 Thevathasan, W., Coyne, T.J., Hyam, J.A. *et al.* (2011) Pedunculopontine nucleus stimulation improves gait freezing in Parkinson disease. *Neurosurgery*, **69**, 1248-1253.

18 Giladi, N. & Nieuwboer, A. (2008) Understanding and treating freezing of gait in Parkinsonism, proposed working definition, and setting the stage. *Movement Disorders*, **23**, S423-S425.

19 Zrinzo, L., Zrinzo, L.V., Tisch, S. *et al.* (2008) Stereotactic localization of the human pedunculopontine nucleus: atlas-based coordinates and validation of magnetic resonance imaging protocol for direct localization. *Brain: A Journal of Neurology*, **131**, 1588-1598.

20 Yelnik, J. (2007) PPN or PPD, what is the target for deep brain stimulation in Parkinson's disease. *Brain: A Journal of Neurology*, **130**, e79.

21 Schallenbrand, C. & Wahren, W. (1977) *Atlas for Stereotaxy of the Human Brain*. George Thieme, Stuttgart.
22 Ferraye, M.U., Gerardin, P., Debu, B. *et al.* (2009) Pedunculopontine nucleus stimulation induces monocular oscillopsia. *Journal of Neurology, Neurosurgery, and Psychiatry*, **80**, 228-231.
23 Jenkinson, N., Brittain, J.S., Hicks, S.L. *et al.* (2012) On the origin of oscillopsia during pedunculopontine stimulation. *Stereotactic and Functional Neurosurgery*, **90**, 124-129.

Chapter 6

Deep Brain Stimulation in Tremor

Antonios Mammis[1] and Michael Schulder[2]

[1]University of Medicine and Dentistry of New Jersey, New Jersey Medical School, Newark, New Jersey, USA
[2]LIJ School of Medicine, New York, New York, USA

Introduction

Deep brain stimulation (DBS) is a non-destructive, reversible, and programmable method of treating a number of neurologic and psychiatric conditions, including tremor. Stimulation of the ventral intermediate nucleus (Vim) of the thalamus for the treatment of essential tremor and parkinsonian tremor was given approval by the Food and Drug Administration (FDA) in 1997. Nowadays, parkinsonian tremor is more commonly treated by stimulating the subthalamic nucleus (STN) and globus pallidus pars interna (GPi). Tremor associated with multiple sclerosis (MS) can also be treated with thalamic stimulation. In contrast to previous methods used to treat tremor surgically, DBS is a non-destructive, reversible, and programmable therapy, whose goal is functional restoration. The exact means by which DBS works in tremor is not known, although it is thought that the various movement disorders and psychiatric disorders treated with DBS represent states of disordered neurophysiologic circuitry. DBS is a means of providing a regular, controlled electrical input to a disturbed circuit to override it. The success of DBS depends largely on patient selection, reasonable expectations, preoperative surgical planning, precise surgical implantation, initial programming, and long-term management.

Neurostimulation: Principles and Practice, First Edition. Edited by Sam Eljamel and Konstantin V. Slavin.
© 2013 John Wiley & Sons, Ltd. Published 2013 by John Wiley & Sons, Ltd.

Patient selection

Essential tremor (ET), Parkinson's disease (PD) tremor, and MS tremor are conditions that pose challenges to conventional medical management, and may become medication refractory. ET is characterized by bilateral action tremor of the hands and forearms, but it may also present with isolated head tremor. Except for the cogwheel phenomenon, there is typically absence of other neurologic signs. There is usually a positive family history, it is of long duration, and there is often a beneficial response to alcohol consumption [1].

Evaluation by a movement disorder neurologist is critical, as up to 50% of patients with ET are misdiagnosed [2]. When the diagnosis has been established, medical management should be optimized. Propranolol and primidone are the mainstay of treatment, but medical management is effective in only 30–70% of patients, and side effects are common [1]. DBS should be considered in the patient with ET whose tremor impairs feeding, using a spoon, using a cup, hygiene, writing, typing, or occupational tasks, and who has failed conventional medical management [1].

PD tremor is classically described as a 3–5 Hz resting, pill-rolling tremor, and is one of the manifestations of PD which can be effectively managed with DBS. Establishing the diagnosis of PD by a movement disorder neurologist is the first step in patient selection. Since there are a number of mimics of idiopathic PD, including dementia with Lewy bodies, vascular parkinsonism, multiple system atrophy, and progressive supranuclear palsy, it is best to wait 3–5 years from the time of diagnosis before considering DBS. Once the diagnosis of PD is made firmly, then it is important to consider the patient's motor symptoms using the Unified Parkinson's Disease Rating Scale (UPDRS) Motor Subscale (Part III) [3]. Tremor, bradykinesia, rigidity, and motor fluctuations generally improve with DBS. Hypophonia, dysphagia, micrographia, freezing, balance problems, cognitive dysfunction, and dysautonomia generally do not improve with DBS. Furthermore, patients should undergo medical optimization prior to consideration of DBS. While the pharmacologic treatment of PD is beyond the scope of this chapter, it is important to understand that the extent of dopaminergic responsiveness is typically predictive of how motor symptoms will respond to DBS [4]. One notable exception, though, is tremor, which is known to often respond better to DBS than maximal medical therapy.

Dementia is common in PD patients and is a symptom that will not improve with DBS. Demented patients usually have difficulty tolerating the operation, and may experience a transient worsening of their cognitive status postoperatively. The Mattis Dementia Rating Scale is helpful in patient selection, and patients with a score less than 120–130 out of 144 are typically excluded [5]. PD patients are prone to depression and should be evaluated preoperatively with a depression scale, such as the Beck Depression Inventory (BDI), or the Montgomery and Asberg Depression Rating Scale (MADRS). Patients with a BDI score greater than 15 or a MADRS score of 7–19 should be excluded [5]. While there is no upper age limit for DBS, the patient's overall health needs to be considered.

Tremor can be found in up to 58% of patients with MS and is a source of significant disability in these patients. This tremor is typically postural, with a frequency of 2.5–7 Hz. Stimulation of Vim thalamus is sometimes utilized for the treatment of medication-refractory MS tremor, but its effectiveness is variable [6]. In a recent study by Torres *et al.* [7], five of 10 patients implanted demonstrated tremor reduction at 1 year postoperatively. At 3-year follow-up, three of the five patients reported continued benefit from stimulation. This fallout is likely due to the progressive nature of MS, as well as the physiologic complexity of MS tremor. Vim DBS may be offered, with caution, to patients with MS.

Rationale for targets

Once an appropriate patient has been selected for DBS, there must be careful surgical planning. For the patient with ET, the Vim nucleus of the thalamus is the target. For patients with PD tremor, the optimal targets are the STN, or GPi. Vim can also be targeted for PD tremor, but we would not expect it to ameliorate any of the other motor symptoms associated with PD.

In preparation for surgical planning, a magnetic resonance imaging (MRI) scan of the brain is obtained prior to implantation. This study is usually obtained while the patient is under sedation in order to minimize motion artifact. Axial and coronal cuts are obtained in both T_2-weighted, and T_1-weighted, contrasted, spoiled gradient echo (SPGR) sequences. Planning software is then used to create image fusion (Figure 6.1), and the targets are selected relative to a point equidistant from the anterior commissure (AC) and posterior commissure (PC), where the mid-sagittal plane intersects the AC–PC plane.

Vim is the target most commonly used for ET, and there is an extensive neurosurgical history dating to the 1950s on this target. Prior to DBS, Vim was the target lesioned in thalamotomy for tremor, but it was noted that high-rate stimulation of this target, prior to lesioning, led to diminishment of the tremor. Vim receives cerebellar afferents, and is located just anterior to the ventralis caudalis nucleus, which receives sensory afferents from the medial lemniscus, and just posterior to the ventralis oralis posterior nucleus, which receives pallidal input [8]. The stereotactic coordinates of the Vim are variable, but can be approximated as $x = 11.5$ mm lateral to lateral wall of the third ventricle, $y =$ the point that bisects the line from the PC to the mid-commissural point, and $z =$ the AC–PC plane.

The STN is commonly targeted for the treatment of PD. The STN is part of the indirect basal ganglia movement circuit, and has connections with the globus pallidus, and SNr. There is a somatotopic organization of the STN, with the dorsolateral aspect being involved with simple voluntary move-

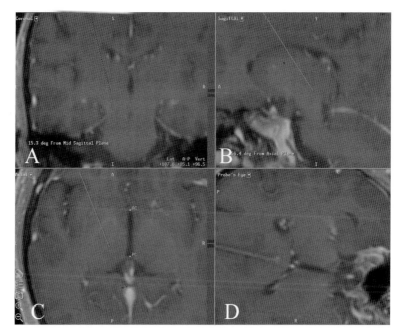

Figure 6.1 Stereotactic planning for deep brain stimulation of the left ventral intermediate nucleus, demonstrating the target and trajectory in the coronal (A), sagittal (B), and axial (C) planes. A probe's eye view (D) can be used to follow the path of the trajectory, in order to plan for a safe corridor.

ments, arranged with face lateral to arm, which is lateral to leg [9]. The stereotactic coordinate that we use are $x = \pm 12$ mm, $y = -4$ mm, and $z = -5$ mm on a coordinate system where [0,0,0] = the point of intersection of the mid-sagittal plane, the AC–PC plane, and the coronal plane which bisects the AC–PC line (Figure 6.2). The rationale of selecting the STN was discussed in Chapter 3.

The GPi is also targeted for PD, or for primary dystonia, and its origins can be traced to pallidotomy procedures. The GPi is involved in both the direct and indirect basal ganglia pathways, and has connections with striatum, STN, and thalamus. The GPi has a somatotopic organization, with the leg located dorsal to arm, which is dorsal to face [9]. The stereotactic coordinates for the GPi are $x = \pm 20$ mm, $y = 2$ mm, and $z = -4$ mm. The rationale for the GPi was discussed in Chapter 4.

After selection of the target, a trajectory is planned. It is helpful to use the SPGR sequence when planning the trajectory while reviewing a probe's eye view. Care must be taken to plan a trajectory which starts anterior to the coronal suture, avoids cortical veins and sulci, avoids the ventricles, and avoids the head of the caudate nucleus. On the day of surgery, a stereotactic frame is placed on the patient, and computed tomography (CT) is performed. The CT is then fused with the pre-planned MRI, and the stereotactic coordinates for the frame are calculated. The details of the surgical technique, as

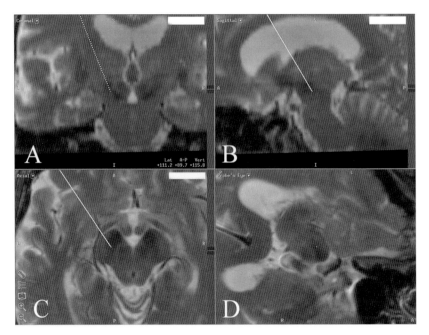

Figure 6.2 Stereotactic planning for deep brain stimulation of the left subthalamic nucleus, demonstrating the target and trajectory in the coronal (A), sagittal (B), and axial (C) planes. A probe's eye view (D) can be used to follow the path of the trajectory, in order to plan for a safe corridor.

well as microelectrode recording, are beyond the scope of this chapter. The implantable pulse generator (IPG) is implanted after implantation of the DBS lead either on the same day or thereafter on a separate day, while initial programming of the device occurs at least 2 weeks after implantation of the leads.

Device programming and patient assessment

The initial programming session is an intense session between patient and programmer, where efficacy and tolerance are evaluated. Ideally, the patient should undergo initial programming while off relevant medications, in order to maximize the tremor. The device is then interrogated, and impedances are checked. The device is then turned on and monopolar (pulse generator case (C) acts as the anode) programming commences, sequentially studying each of the four lead contacts. At each lead contact, the patient is evaluated at progressively increasing amplitudes while evaluating the status of the tremor and observing for any untoward side effects, such as persistent paresthesias, muscle contractions, slurring of speech, visual deficits, and dyskinesias. A comparison of the efficacy of the therapy with the emergence of untoward side effects gives the clinician the physiologic clues to pinpoint the precise anatomic location of the lead. The clinician will then select a monopolar setting based on the contact that yields the best overall balance of efficacy and tolerability. The initially selected amplitude is typically low (just at the threshold of efficacy) to prevent dyskinesias once the patient takes his medications. The pulse width, or duration of each pulse delivered, is variable, and most programmers will select either 60 or 90 μs. The rate, or the number of pulses per second, is typically 130 Hz or greater for PD or ET [9]. After an initial program is selected, the patient is allowed to take his/her medications, and is observed for one or more hours for the development of dyskinesias.

Subsequent to the initial programming, the patient may undergo one or more additional programming sessions to fine-tune the therapy. Additional unipolar programming can be attempted, or bipolar programming can be commenced in order to minimize stimulation-related side effects. In bipolar programming, the lead contacts are designated as anodes and cathodes, which results in a tighter sphere of energy. Programming groups may also be attempted to optimize therapy. Certain patients find that they require different program configurations for different times of the day, or with different activities. By programming different groups, the patient is able to toggle between different programs, using his/her individual programmer. The physician can also allow the patient to self-adjust therapy amplitude within a predetermined range. Finally, in the most challenging cases, the physician can introduce program interleaving. Interleaving allows for automatic, rapid cycling between two different programs. If there is a program which has excellent symptomatic relief, but which has some troublesome side effects, sometimes cycling that with another program with less effective symptomatic relief, but without side effects, will yield excellent symptomatic relief and no side effects.

Assessment and evidence

The evidence for the efficacy of DBS for ET and PD tremor is robust. Tremor in ET is formally evaluated using the Fahn-Tolosa-Marin tremor rating scale. It is also helpful to evaluate handwriting samples, or spiral drawings with stimulation off and then on (Figure 6.3).

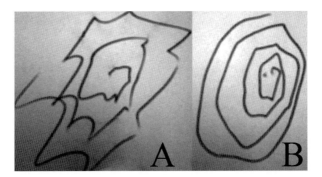

Figure 6.3 Spiral drawings from a patient with essential tremor who underwent placement of bilateral ventral intermediate nucleus deep brain stimulation (DBS) leads with DBS turned off (A), and then turned on (B).

There have been myriad studies since 1997 demonstrating significant improvement in hand tremor (ranging from 50% to 91%) and activities of daily living (ADLs) (36-86%) [9,10]. PD is assessed with the UPDRS, and there have been multiple studies showing the benefit on Vim, STN, and GPi stimulation on parkinsonian tremor. The multicentre European study of thalamic stimulation in parkinsonian and essential tremor found a 90% tremor reduction in patients with PD [10]. Vim stimulation did not yield significant improvement in rigidity or ADLs. STN and GPi stimulation in PD have both demonstrated consistent improvements in tremor, rigidity, bradykinesia, dyskinesia, and overall quality of life. With GPi stimulation, off-period parkinsonism has been shown to improve by 30-50%, while on-period parkinsonism improves up to 25%. STN stimulation yields 45-65% improvement in off-period parkinsonism, and 67-83% improvement in on-period parkinsonism [11].

Complications

Complications of DBS surgery include intracranial hemorrhage or stroke. These are uncommon, and very rarely result in permanent neurologic deficit. Infection, especially at the IPG site, is a potential complication, with rates varying by institution and by implanter. An infection of the DBS system is usually not dangerous to the patient, but should be treated by explanting the device. Preoperative screening of patients for meticillin-resistant *Staphylococcus aureus* (MRSA) colonization can help diminish infection rates. Patients who have MRSA colonization should undergo a course of oral and intranasal antibiotics to eradicate the colonization prior to implantation. Transient cognitive decline is sometimes encountered in elderly patients who undergo bilateral stage I procedures or who have leads that traverse the caudate head. In our experience, this problem can be avoided by staging lead implantations by at least 3 months' duration. Finally, there is the potential for therapy-related complications which are dependent on lead position. These potential untoward side effects are summarized in Table 6.1.

Table 6.1 Clinical effects of deep brain stimulation lead placement

Lead position	VIM	STN	GPi
Too anterior	N/A	Contractions; Dysarthria	N/A
Too posterior	Paresthesias	Paresthesias	Contractions; Dysarthria
Too medial	N/A	Paresthesias; Diplopia; Mood changes	Contractions; Dysarthria
Too lateral	Contractions; Dysarthria	Contractions; Dysarthria	N/A
Too superior	N/A	N/A	N/A
Too inferior	N/A	Mood changes	Visual phenomena

Conclusions

DBS for ET or PD tremor is a safe, effective, FDA-approved and CE-marked therapy. The Vim thalamic nucleus is the most commonly used target in ET, while the STN or GPi are mostly used in PD. Advances in stereotactic targeting systems and in pulse generator technology have made implantation and management of this therapy more efficient and more powerful. Fundamentally, though, the success of DBS depends largely on patient selection, reasonable expectations, preoperative surgical planning, precise surgical implantation, tailored programming, and careful long-term management.

Further reading

Bakay, R.A.E. (ed.) (2009) *Movement Disorder Surgery: The Essentials.* Thieme, New York.

Lozano, A.M., Gildenberg, P.L. & Tasker, R.R. (eds) (2009) *Textbook of Stereotactic and Functional Neurosurgery,* 2nd ed. Springer, Berlin.

Marks, W.J. (ed.) (2011) *Deep Brain Stimulation Management.* Cambridge, New York.

Starr, P.A., Barbaro, N.M. & Larson, P.S. (eds) (2009) *Neurosurgical Operative Atlas, Functional Neurosurgery,* 2nd ed. Thieme, New York.

References

1 Benito-Leon, J. & Louis, E.D. (2007) *Clinical update: diagnosis and treatment of essential tremor. Lancet,* **369**, 1152-1154.

2 Jain, S., Lo, S.E. & Louis, E.D. (2006) *Common misdiagnosis of a common neurologic disorder: how are we misdiagnosing essential tremor? Archives of Neurology,* **63**, 1100-1104.

3 Fahn, S. & Elton, R.L. (1987) Members of the UPDRS development committee. United Parkinson's Disease Rating Scale. In: S. Fahn, C.D. Marsden, C.B. Calne & M. Goldstien (eds), *Recent developments in Parkinson's Disease,* pp. 153-163. MacMillan Healthcare Information, Florham Park.

4 Charles, P.D., Van Blercom, N., Krack, P. et al. (2002) *Predictors of effective bilateral subthalamic nucleus stimulation for PD. Neurology,* **59**, 932-934.

5 Defer, G.L., Widner, H., Marie, R.M. et al. (1999) *Core assessment program for surgical interventional therapies in Parkinson's disease (CAPSIT-PD). Movement Disorders,* **14**, 572-584.

6 Schulder, M., Sernas, T.J. & Karimi, R. (2003) *Thalamic stimulation in patients with multiple sclerosis: long-term follow-up. Stereotactic and Functional Neurosurgery,* **80** (1-4), 48-55.

7 Torres, C.V., Moro, E., Lopez-Rios, A.L. et al. (2010) *Deep brain stimulation of the ventral intermediate nucleus of the thalamus for tremor in patients with multiple sclerosis. Neurosurgery,* **67** (3), 646-651.

8 Hassler, R. (1982) Architectonic organization of the thalamic nuclei. In: G. Schaltenbrand & A. Walker (eds), *Stereotaxy of Human Brain,* pp. 140-180. Thieme, New York.

9 Marks, W.J. (ed.) (2011) *Deep Brain Stimulation Management*. Cambridge, New York.

10 Limousin, P., Speelman, J.D., Gielen, F. & Janssens, M. (1999) *Multicentre European study of thalamic stimulation in parkinsonian and essential tremor.* Journal of Neurology, Neurosurgery, and Psychiatry, **66**, 289-296.

11 The deep brain stimulation for Parkinson's Disease Study Group (2001) *Deep brain stimulation of the subthalamic nucleus or the pars interna of the globus pallidus in Parkinson's disease. The New England Journal of Medicine*, **345**, 956-963.

Chapter 7

Deep Brain Stimulation in Dystonia

Ludvic Zrinzo

UCL Institute of Neurology, University College London, and National Hospital for Neurology and Neurosurgery, London, UK

Introduction

Dystonia is defined as abnormally sustained muscle contraction, usually producing twisting and repetitive movements or abnormal postures. Three criteria are usually considered for classification purposes: age of symptom onset, body region affected (focal, segmental, or generalized), and underlying etiology (primary, heredodegenerative, or secondary).

Numerous distinct pathophysiological mechanisms may result in dystonia, making it the third most common movement disorder in humans. Dystonia may follow macroscopic damage to a variety of brain regions, most commonly of the basal ganglia and thalamus, brainstem, and cerebellum. Genetic insults may also give rise to dystonia with numerous monogenetic loci (DYT) being defined in the last few decades. DYT mutations have variable penetrance and may give rise to one of three phenotypes: primary dystonia, dystonia plus (with additional signs such as parkinsonism or myoclonus), and paroxysmal forms of dystonia/dyskinesia. Abnormalities of neural connectivity, plasticity, or synaptic regulation at the cellular level can result in dystonia. Impaired inhibition, aberrant cortical plasticity, and abnormal sensory processing are the neurophysiologic hallmarks of dystonia.

Pharmacological treatment of dystonia is often inadequate or associated with undesirable side effects. However, notable exceptions include dopa-responsive dystonia and chemodenervation with botulinum toxin in some focal dystonia.

Surgical therapies include peripheral denervation and functional stereotactic surgery. In the 1960s and 1970s ablative surgery targeting the thalamus

Neurostimulation: Principles and Practice, First Edition. Edited by Sam Eljamel and Konstantin V. Slavin.
© 2013 John Wiley & Sons, Ltd. Published 2013 by John Wiley & Sons, Ltd.

and pallidum were used in patients with intractable dystonia, probably after surgical pioneers noted the beneficial effect of surgery on dystonia within the context of Parkinson's disease (PD). Thalamotomy (ventralis oralis anterior and posterior nucleus: Voa–Vop) is still employed by some groups with favorable outcomes. Early reports of intermittent stimulation of deep-seated structures were limited by technical challenges. However, the evolution of surgery for dystonia has paralleled that of PD and, following early reports in 1999, deep brain stimulation (DBS) has all but replaced ablative stereotactic procedures in contemporary practice.

Target and rationale

The posteroventral pallidum has emerged as the most popular target for DBS in the management of dystonia. A multicenter French study of pallidal DBS in primary generalized and segmental dystonia randomly allocated patients to a double-blind cross-over study 3 months after surgery [1]. Patients underwent evaluation in the presence and absence of neurostimulation. Raters blinded to stimulation state confirmed significantly better mean dystonia motor scores with stimulation. At 3-year follow-up, mean motor improvements of 58% from baseline were documented in these patients [2]. A class I German multicenter study randomized patients with generalized and segmental dystonia to receive active or sham stimulation for the first 3 months after pallidal DBS [3]. Blinded raters, assessing dystonia severity from videotape review, confirmed significantly greater motor improvement in stimulated patients. The positive effect of pallidal DBS on several types of dystonia is further supported by a large number of reports from different centers. A smaller number of open-label studies reported beneficial effects on dystonia with DBS at other brain targets including the subthalamic nucleus (STN), ventral intermediate nucleus, and Voa–Vop nuclei of the thalamus.

Assessment scales

Numerous dystonia scales have been employed to assess specific types of dystonia [4]. The two most commonly employed scales are the Burke-Fahn-Marsden dystonia rating scale (BFM) and the Toronto Western Spasmodic Torticollis Rating Scale (TWSTRS).

The BFM is the most widely used scale in studies of DBS for generalized dystonia, has been validated, and enjoys a good interrater and retest reliability. The BFM is divided into two parts: the movement scale and the disability scale. The movement score ranges from 0 to 120, where zero represents no dystonia, and is the sum of body regions items. The total disability score ranges from 0 to 30 and is the sum of scores for seven functional items rated 0-4, except walking, which has a maximal severity score of 6.

The TWSTRS is a validated scale that focuses on the clinical features of cervical dystonia and is widely used in clinical reports. It includes a videotape protocol that allows assessment of patients in a standardized fashion. Six domains are examined with a maximal severity score of 35.

Clinical studies often employ additional scales to assess the impact of therapy on quality of life.

Referral criteria and patient selection

Dystonia may present in myriad ways and may be dismissed as a psychological problem by the uninitiated. A movement disorder neurologist should review patients with an unusual or unexplained movement disorder. Patients with a diagnosis of medically refractory dystonia should then be referred to an experienced multidisciplinary DBS team for further assessment.

A detailed history and examination is complemented by appropriate investigations that include structural magnetic resonance imaging (MRI) of the brain, neuropsychological evaluation, and formal assessment of dystonia using appropriate standardized scales as discussed above.

The huge range of clinical presentations, variations in study design, surgical practice, and programming techniques make predictions of outcome in an individual patient extremely challenging. Nevertheless, previous reports do provide insight into the likely outcome after DBS surgery in dystonia.

Motor features and associated pain in primary generalized and segmental dystonia are potentially responsive to globus pallidus pars interna (GPi) DBS. Primary forms of dystonia and tardive dystonia tend to respond well to pallidal DBS, especially when surgery is performed at an early stage after symptom onset and in patients with less severe disability. Moreover, DYT-1 positive dystonia tends to respond better than DYT-1 negative ones, where outcome can be very heterogeneous. The presence of fixed skeletal deformities appears to be associated with a lower degree of improvement. Larger internal pallidum volume, as defined on MRI, has been associated with better clinical response to DBS in patients with primary dystonia [5].

Cervical dystonia (spasmodic torticollis) responds well to pallidal DBS in both blinded and open-label series. The results of pallidal DBS for Meige syndrome also compare favorably to other forms of focal or segmental dystonia, as do the results of smaller series of patients with myoclonus dystonia. A smaller number of patients with cervical dystonia, Meige syndrome, or myoclonus dystonia have undergone STN DBS with good effect.

A limited number of patients with dystonia in the context of Lubag (DYT-3) and myoclonus dystonia suggest a positive and consistent response to pallidal DBS, especially on the mobile components of dystonia. Patients with tardive dystonia also seem to respond well to GPi DBS. Other forms of secondary dystonia have a variable response to such surgery. Patients severely affected by "cerebral palsy," with a mixed clinical picture of dystonia and spasticity, present a particular challenge. Even minimal improvement on dystonia rating scales in well-selected patients may facilitate nursing care and have a valuable impact on quality of life.

Pallidal DBS in heredodegenerative conditions (e.g., Huntington's disease or pantothenate kinase-associated neurodegeneration) can offer some improvement in motor scores and pain, but there is no evidence that it benefits associated non-motor symptoms or that it alters the underlying degenerative process.

Brain MRI, to confirm diagnosis and assess structural abnormalities, is an important investigation in the preoperative selection process. Screening for psychiatric comorbidities is recommended. Although psychiatric complications are rare after pallidal DBS, severe premorbid psychiatric symptoms may represent a contraindication to surgery. As with any DBS procedure, increasing age and a history of hypertension are risk factors for hemorrhagic complications.

DBS in dystonia may be expected to reduce the severity of motor impairment and pain, thereby improving quality of life and activities of daily living (ADLs). Patients and their families should be informed that the full benefit of DBS in dystonia might be delayed for weeks or months. It has been proposed that synaptic plasticity must occur in response to the induced orthodromic and antidromic activation before full symptomatic benefit can be achieved. This is supported by the observation that some dystonic symptoms may take a variable amount of time to recur after cessation of stimulation.

Hardware choice must be adapted to the particular patient. Dual channel, primary cell, implantable pulse generators (IPGs) are available when performing bilateral lead implants. Nevertheless, some centers advocate the use of two single channel IPGs, especially in patients with severe axial dystonia. This approach reduces the risk of complete cessation of stimulation and the potential for severe life-threatening dystonic rebound with IPG failure. Rechargeable IPGs may offer significant advantages in suitable patients, especially since a higher current drain is often used in dystonic conditions.

DBS may be considered a safe, effective surgical treatment for medically refractory dystonia. However, surgery must be tailored to the individual patient, the potential benefits and hazards considered and patient expectations managed appropriately prior to surgery.

Surgical procedure

The optimal target within the internal pallidum has not been determined with certainty. However, there appears to be a consensus that the target point is the posteroventrolateral sensorimotor portion, similar to the pallidal target in PD. One study suggests that leads located in the most posterior and ventral part of this region provide the greatest clinical improvement [6].

The traditional surgical approach relies on ventricular landmarks to estimate the location of deep-seated anatomical structures such as the pallidum. The indirect atlas-defined coordinates for the pallidal target are approximately 21mm lateral, 2mm anterior, and 5mm inferior to the midcommissural point. Surrogate markers that rely on the expert interpretation of physiological or clinical observations are often employed to "refine" intraoperative targeting. This approach requires multiple brain penetrations and may necessitate surgery under local anesthesia. Although microelectrode recording (MER) techniques are widely used, good outcomes have been described with and without MER. Teams using MER should be aware that the external and internal pallidum exhibit similar neuronal activity, that general anesthesia may further hinder interpretation of neuronal activity, and that the use of MER has been associated with a higher risk of hemorrhage.

MRI-guided and MRI-verified targeting provides an alternative and increasingly popular surgical approach. Appropriate stereotactic MRI sequences capitalize on the ability to localize the pallidal architecture directly in individual patients. The resulting radiological anatomy enables direct targeting, confirms access, and guides relocation should it be required. Moreover, systematic analysis of targeting errors permits the calibration of target coordinates during subsequent procedures, thus tending to minimize the number of brain penetrations [7]. This approach also allows surgery to be performed under general anesthesia, an important practical consideration when performing surgery on children or other patients with severe dystonia or associated disabilities.

A number of published MRI protocols allow clear visualization of pallidal architecture in individual patients. A modified proton density MR sequence for targeting the posteroventral pallidum at 1.5T is shown in Figure 7.1 [8].

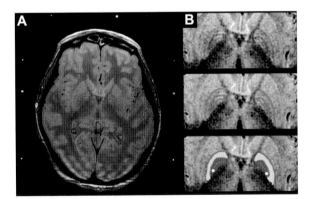

Figure 7.1 Neuroanatomy of the lentiform nucleus and magnetic resonance imaging (MRI) correlates (A) stereotactic axial proton density MRI at the anterior commissure–posterior commissure (AC-PC) level. B, Detail from MRI scan clearly demonstrates the three laminae, outlined in red in the middle panel (from lateral to medial: the lateral, medial, and accessory medullary lamina). The external pallidum is yellow and the internal pallidum blue in the lower panel with a white dot depicting the "motor" pallidal target at the level of the AC-PC plane. Refer to color plate section for color version of this figure.

The putamen, internal, and external pallidum and the pallidocapsular border can easily be seen at the level of the anterior commissure. Commercially available software facilitates the planning of a surgical trajectory to the posteroventral pallidal target that lies 4–5 mm inferior to this plane and immediately superior and lateral to the optic tract.

Programming parameters

DBS programming in patients with dystonia differs substantially from that in patients with tremor or PD. The beneficial "micro-lesion" effect, often present before starting stimulation after DBS for other movement disorders, may not be present or is much less prominent after DBS for dystonia. In addition, improvement of dystonic symptoms in response to stimulation is often delayed by hours or days with gradual progression of benefit over several months. As a result, DBS programming in dystonia requires patience from both patient and physician.

Practice differs between different centers with stimulation commencing from days to 1 month postoperatively. Screening of contacts in monopolar mode may determine the threshold for acute stimulation-induced adverse effects (e.g., capsular effects, visual flashes) that could limit the therapeutic window. There are no evidence-based guidelines to DBS programming in dystonia. Although most groups commence with monopolar stimulation of the deepest contact, others favor bipolar stimulation with adjacent contacts. A wide variation in stimulation parameters exists, especially in pulse width (60–450 μs). Most centers use frequencies of 130 Hz and above but some reports have reported additional benefit with a lower frequency of 60 Hz. Pragmatic algorithms on how to approach DBS programming in dystonia are available in the published literature [9].

Complications, side effects, monitoring, and troubleshooting

Positive outcomes after DBS for dystonia are widely reported with published evidence extending up to 10 years [10]. Once optimal stimulation parameters are defined there is usually little need for further modification in the following years.

Failure to improve dystonia requires an assessment of whether the DBS leads are well located. This underscores the importance of obtaining appropriate imaging following surgery, preferably stereotactic MRI using a sequence that adequately demonstrates the relevant anatomy (Figure 7.2). Several programming strategies may be adopted if patients present with a persistent low threshold for capsular or visual side effects (such as bipolar or interleaving stimulation), but lead relocation may be required if such efforts fail to resolve matters. Exceptional cases describe more improvement in secondary dystonia with thalamic than with pallidal DBS.

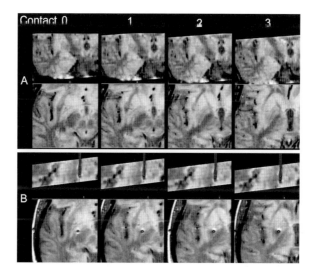

Figure 7.2 Pallidal deep brain stimulation: stereotactic planning and verification of contact location. Stereotactic proton density magnetic resonance images. A, Preoperative coronal (above) and axial (below) views. A trajectory that maximizes the number of contacts within the posteroventral pallidum was planned. The center-to-center distance between the quadripolar electrode contacts is 2 mm (Model 3389 DBS lead, Medtronic®, Minneapolis, MN). Each panel demonstrates the planned stereotactic coordinates (in green) and location for each contact (small red dot), from contact 0 through 3. Contact 0 was planned to lie just superior and lateral to the lateral border of the optic tract, an oblique oval hypointense structure in coronal section and a hypointense band running from anteromedial to posterolateral on axial images. The lateral and medial medullary laminae can be identified on all four coronal images. On axial images, the medullary laminae are only seen with clarity at the level of contacts 2 and 3. The accessory medullary lamina can be visualized on some of the axial and coronal sections as a thin hypointense line bisecting the internal pallidum. B, Postoperative trajectory views (above) and axial views (below). The implanted electrode produces a signal void artifact that is larger than the actual electrode dimensions. A targeting error of 1.0 mm accounts for the difference between the planned location of each contact in the axial images in row A and the actual location of each contact in the axial images in row B. Contacts 0, 1, and 2 lie within the posterolateral internal pallidum whereas contact 3 lies in the internal medullary lamina. Refer to color plate section for color version of this figure.

As with any DBS procedure, patients and carers should be educated as to the signs of early and delayed infection and the importance of seeking early expert advice. Management of hardware infection can be more challenging in dystonia patients than in those with PD, since rebound of symptoms cannot be mitigated as effectively with increases in medication. Some centers have suggested maintaining stimulation by externalizing the IPG and distal portion of the cables while using antibiotics to eradicate infection of an abdominal IPG pocket. Others have reported ablation via an implanted lead before removal of the hardware.

The incidence of relapse secondary to hardware failure was initially thought to be higher in dystonia than in other DBS indications; however, this observation has been challenged in more recent studies, probably by widespread adoption of simple surgical precautions that lower the risk of hardware failure (e.g., ensuring that lead to cable connectors do not migrate down into the neck). Sudden cessation of stimulation in patients with severe dystonia may become a medical emergency and is best avoided by anticipating the IPG replacement before the natural "end of life."

Stimulation-induced side effects of pallidal DBS include speech abnormalities (dysarthria, dysphonia) and can often be addressed by adjustment of stimulation settings. Pallidal DBS may sometimes elicit features of parkinsonism (freezing of gait and slowness of movement) that are completely reversible on stopping stimulation. Selection of more dorsal contacts may also help minimize such symptoms. There is no evidence that pallidal DBS can cause psychiatric side effects; however, rare reports of suicide after pallidal DBS have occurred in patients with psychiatric problems that predated surgery.

With longer-term follow-up, a subset of patients may exhibit a relapse in symptoms, either due to stimulation tolerance or progression of the underlying pathology. The Montpellier group has reported that placement of an additional lead in the posteroventral pallidum may be of benefit in such patients with primary generalized dystonia. Conversely, there are rare reports of patients whose dystonic symptoms do not return after cessation of chronic stimulation.

Conclusions

Pallidal DBS can significantly improve motor scores and quality of life in well-selected patients with dystonia. A multidisciplinary approach by a dedicated functional neurosurgery team that places an emphasis on patient safety and life long follow-up is required to achieve the best possible clinical results.

Further reading

Andrews, C., Aviles-Olmos, I., Hariz, M.I. & Foltynie, T. (2010) *Which patients with dystonia benefit from deep brain stimulation? A metaregression of individual patient outcomes. Journal of Neurology, Neurosurgery, and Psychiatry*, **81** (12), 1383-1389.

Breakefield, X.O., Blood, A.J., Li, Y. et al. (2008) *The pathophysiological basis of dystonias. Nature Reviews. Neuroscience*, **9** (3), 222-234.

Bronte-Stewart, H., Taira, T., Valldeoriola, F. et al. (2011) *Inclusion and exclusion criteria for DBS in dystonia. Movement Disorders*, **26**, S5-S16.

References

1 Vidailhet, M., Vercueil, L., Houeto, J.-L. *et al.* (2005) *Bilateral deep-brain stimulation of the globus pallidus in primary generalized dystonia. The New England Journal of Medicine*, **352** (5), 459–467.

2 Vidailhet, M., Vercueil, L., Houeto, J.-L. *et al.* (2007) *Bilateral, pallidal, deep-brain stimulation in primary generalised dystonia: a prospective 3 year follow-up study. The Lancet Neurology.*, **6** (3), 223–229.

3 Kupsch, A., Benecke, R., Müller, J. *et al.* (2006) *Pallidal deep-brain stimulation in primary generalized or segmental dystonia. The New England Journal of Medicine*, **355** (19), 1978–1990.

4 Thobois, S., Taira, T., Comella, C. *et al.* (2011) *Pre-operative evaluations for DBS in dystonia. Movement Disorders*, **26** (Suppl. 1), S17–S22.

5 Vasques, X., Cif, L., Hess, O. *et al.* (2009) *Prognostic value of globus pallidus internus volume in primary dystonia treated by deep brain stimulation. Journal of Neurosurgery*, **110** (2), 220–228.

6 Tisch, S., Zrinzo, L., Limousin, P. *et al.* (2007) *Effect of electrode contact location on clinical efficacy of pallidal deep brain stimulation in primary generalised dystonia. Journal of Neurology, Neurosurgery, and Psychiatry*, **78** (12), 1314–1319.

7 Holl, E.M., Petersen, E.A., Foltynie, T. *et al.* (2010) *Improving targeting in image-guided frame-based deep brain stimulation. Neurosurgery*, **67** (2 Suppl. Operative), 437–447.

8 Hirabayashi, H., Tengvar, M. & Hariz, M.I. (2002) *Stereotactic imaging of the pallidal target. Movement Disorders*, **17** (S3), S130–S134.

9 Kupsch, A., Tagliati, M., Vidailhet, M. *et al.* (2011) *Early postoperative management of DBS in dystonia: programming, response to stimulation, adverse events, medication changes, evaluations, and troubleshooting. Movement Disorders*, **26** (Suppl. 1), S37–S53.

10 Cif, L., Vasques, X., Gonzalez, V. *et al.* (2010) *Long-term follow-up of DYT1 dystonia patients treated by deep brain stimulation: an open-label study. Movement Disorders*, **25** (3), 289–299.

Chapter 8

Deep Brain Stimulation in Epilepsy

Michael G. Kaplitt

Weill Cornell Medical College, New York, New York, USA

Introduction

Deep brain stimulation (DBS) has long been used as an effective therapy for movement disorders. In recent years, there has been increasing interest in DBS applications to other areas, particularly those in which stimulation within a target brain region is believed to specifically influence circuits that are critical to the pathophysiology of a given disease. These include major depression, drug addiction, and dementia. Although the mechanisms of DBS action in movement disorders and newer experimental areas remain unclear, the general view is that tonic modulation to either inhibit neuronal firing or to activate fibers that may release inhibitory neurotransmitters can yield significant normalization in the physiology of these dysfunctional circuits.

Epilepsy has long been considered as a surgical disease for those who do not adequately respond to medication. Standard procedures for refractory epilepsy include various forms of temporal lobectomy for those with unilateral mesial temporal sclerosis (MTS), lesionectomy for epilepsy caused by an identifiable focus in a non-eloquent area, corpus callosotomy, functional hemispherectomy in children, and multiple subpial transections [1]. However, a substantial minority of patients either fail to respond to traditional surgery or are not candidates for resective surgery because of an inability to localize the epileptic focus to a single site or because of the eloquent location of a demonstrable focus. In these cases, neuromodulation has been considered, with the first and most widely used form being vagus nerve stimulation (VNS).

Neurostimulation: Principles and Practice, First Edition. Edited by Sam Eljamel and Konstantin V. Slavin.

To more directly address the mechanisms whereby seizures establish and spread through the brain without the need for resective surgery, DBS for epilepsy has gained enthusiasm. This is in part due to the increasing recognition of epilepsy as a network disease, with greater similarities to other diseases of brain networks for which DBS is more routinely considered. Several brain targets have been explored, but the target that has advanced the farthest in clinical practice is the anterior nucleus (AN) of the thalamus. Other targets that have also been tested include the centromedian nucleus (CM) of the thalamus, the subthalamic nucleus (STN), and the amygdala-hippocampus. The overall goal of DBS in epilepsy is to provide a tonic modulation that will act essentially as a sentinel to either prevent abnormal firing from an epileptic focus or to prevent spread and generalization of a seizure and thereby improve quality of life. A more detailed rationale for the use of each target and some details of key surgical methodological points are provided.

Referral criteria

Regardless of the target, many of the major considerations when evaluating a patient for DBS surgery are similar. The benefits (outlined later) and potential risks of surgery, including hemorrhage and infection, generally preclude considering DBS for any patient who has seizures well controlled with medication. It is also generally accepted that patients who are good candidates for resective surgery, such as patients with unilateral MTS or those in whom a discrete, operable seizure focus can be identified by electrophysiological localization, should be encouraged to undergo surgical excision prior to considering other procedures. Patients who would be considered good candidates for DBS include those who have failed to achieve acceptable seizure control following an adequate trial of more than one antiepileptic drug (most studies and practitioners consider failure of three medications to be reasonable) and who either do not have an isolated, resectable seizure focus (including patients with bilateral anterior temporal onset) or who have failed prior resective surgery [2]. Some physicians may consider vagus nerve stimulation (VNS) in this setting, but there is no evidence that patients respond better to VNS than DBS and many of the patients who responded to DBS in the recently reported double-blind study of AN DBS for epilepsy (SANTE trial; see later) had failed prior VNS [3]. Therefore, DBS may be considered as an up-front alternative to VNS in the patients outlined earlier. There is some evidence that patients with Lennox–Gastaut syndrome (LGS), which is a childhood syndrome of daily, multiple seizures of varying types, may respond particularly well to CM DBS (as well as VNS) [4]. Given the presumptive mechanism of DBS to prevent seizure spread and generalization, it is not surprising that patients with simple partial seizures may not respond as well to DBS as patients with complex partial or secondary generalized seizures.

Rationale for deep brain stimulation in epilepsy

Anterior nucleus of the thalamus

The AN is in the center of the circuit of Papez, the classical pathway by which memory information is transmitted through key structures throughout the brain [5]. This begins in the hippocampus, projects through the fornix to the mammillary bodies and via the mammillothalamic tract to the AN, then on to the cingulate gyrus and subsequently to the parahippocampal gyrus and entorhinal cortex, where the circuit is completed with a projection back to the hippocampus. It is believed that seizures spread through this circuit, which results in generalization. Therefore, inhibition or modulation of AN is believed to prevent spread of seizures along this pathway, thereby reducing the rate of more complex or generalized seizures. Animal studies have supported this hypothesis, demonstrating that either lesioning or high-frequency stimulation can either reduce seizures or increase seizure thresholds in various models. These data are consistent with a model of high-frequency stimulation inhibiting AN activity, as is additional data demonstrating that low-frequency AN stimulation lowers seizure thresholds in animals.

Centromedian nucleus of the thalamus

The CM is one of the intralaminar thalamic nuclei within the middle of the thalamus that are widely connected to various brainstem structures as well as to many regions of the cerebral cortex. The CM tends to connect more to sensorimotor territories within the basal ganglia, particularly within the striatum and may be involved in a parallel information processing system for motor function. The adjacent parafascicular (Pf) nucleus, which is often viewed as part of a complex with the CM, is also widely connected but generally to more associative and limbic territories within the basal ganglia and cortex. There also appear to be many intrinsic connections with other thalamic nuclei. Therefore, it is not surprising that stimulation within the CM would also be considered as a potential therapy for epilepsy, to reduce seizure spread that may occur along a variety of brain networks influenced by CM and/or the CM-Pf complex. There have been many open-label small series that have indicated in some cases dramatic efficacy, with 80–90% improvements in seizures. A particular target for CM DBS has been LGS, as outlined earlier, with specific series of these patients demonstrating substantial improvement in seizure frequencies [4]. While CM DBS has not been subjected to the type of large, randomized double-blind study described later for AN DBS, there have been two studies in which small series of patients were randomly assigned to stimulation ON and OFF, and unfortunately both of these have failed to demonstrate a significant effect of active stimulation on primary outcomes [4,6]. However, further investigation has suggested that subsets of patients such as LGS may particularly benefit, and perhaps electrode location may also influence outcome [4]. Given the small numbers of patients in each study, it is difficult to assess with high confidence specific factors, which may influence outcome.

Subthalamic nucleus

The STN is in the middle of the basal ganglia circuit, connecting the external segment of the globus pallidus to the internal segment and the pars reticulata (SNr). Given these connections and the central role of this structure in regulating movement, it has become the most popular target for DBS electrodes in patients with PD. However, the modulation of the SNr has also been shown to influence seizure activity in animals, perhaps through outflow projections to the thalamus, which widely influences brain circuits, and the STN also has direct connections with various cortical sites. Although the potential mechanism of action remains unclear, STN stimulation has been effective in several animal models of epilepsy. There have been several small reports of effective STN DBS for epilepsy, most using stimulation parameters similar to STN DBS for PD (high frequency, low pulse width) although in some cases at higher amplitudes, raising some question as to whether the mechanism of action is due to intrinsic stimulation of the STN proper or due to spread to nearby fibers of passage which widely connect basal ganglia and thalamic structures [2,7,8]. However, all of these studies have essentially been case reports or at best pilots, with very small numbers (two to five patients in most cases) being evaluated in an open-label fashion. It is difficult therefore to generate definitive conclusions regarding the efficacy of STN DBS for epilepsy, or to determine optimal patient selection or programming parameters. However, given the general agreement among these small studies of demonstrable efficacy of STN DBS for epilepsy, larger studies are certainly warranted.

Assessment methods

The optimal assessment method for efficacy of DBS in epilepsy has been a subject of some debate. During programming, assessments are more similar to DBS for dystonia, where there is usually little immediate therapeutic feedback, compared with essential tremor or PD, where positive symptomatic responses are generally used to guide programming. Long term, the most obvious outcome measure is seizure freedom, which is the absence of seizures for a period of time. While the ultimate goal of any epilepsy treatment, complete seizure freedom is very difficult to achieve in the population of patients being considered for DBS. However, a variety of additional assessment methods can be utilized to evaluate efficacy. Reduction in seizure frequency is a commonly used outcome measure. In blinded clinical trials, a significant reduction beyond placebo is generally used, but this is not applicable to general practice. A meaningful reduction in seizure frequency for any individual is difficult to quantify and is somewhat subjective. For several studies, this has translated into a responder rate in which patients are considered responders if they have a certain percentage reduction in seizure frequency from baseline (often greater than 40-50%).

A change in the nature of the seizures should also be monitored. For example, patients may have variable reductions in overall seizure numbers, but can see a shift from more morbid and debilitating complex partial and/or generalized seizures to more tolerable simple partial seizures. Patients may even report ongoing auras but they do not turn into actual seizures as often. This again may reflect a mechanism of DBS which may not directly block the seizure focus but which reduces spread and generalization. Additional assessment methods include quality of life measures, such as return to work or school, and measures for adverse events of DBS, such as depression and cognitive measures. For this reason, patients should be evaluated with formal neuropsychological testing prior to surgery and then again following surgery when stable stimulation parameters are obtained. Unlike PD, medication reduction is usually not a method of assessing efficacy in DBS for epilepsy, since most patients have inadequate responses to medications already and medication effects in epilepsy are usually less linear than in PD.

Evidence level to date

The strongest evidence to date supporting efficacy of DBS for epilepsy derives from studies using AN as the target. A fascinating historical feature of DBS in this particular target is that the first reported human study was performed by Irving Cooper, a pioneer of movement disorders surgery, in 1980, long before the first commercial DBS device was approved for sale for any indication [9]. Of the six patients included in that study, five were reported to have greater than 50% reduction in seizure frequencies following surgery. Following extensive animal studies throughout the 1990s which more strongly supported the validity of this approach, and with the widespread use of commercially available DBS devices for movement disorders surgery, several small pilot studies were performed which supported Cooper's original observation and provided justification for a more extensive trial. A reduction in seizure frequency was also noted simply from electrode insertion prior to initiating stimulation after 4 weeks, consistent with a microlesioning effect observed in movement disorders surgery. Following onset of stimulation, there was no additional improvement in patients in the one study in which this was systematically studied, and in the same study the cessation of stimulation at 7-17 months following surgery for 2 months did not result in a significant decline towards presurgical seizure rates. This raised important questions regarding the mechanism of DBS action and the role of stimulation in the ultimate outcome from DBS insertion.

A large, randomized double-blind study of AN DBS for epilepsy was recently completed to address some remaining questions and to obtain data which could be used to obtain approval for commercialization of this methodology. The Stimulation of the Anterior Nucleus of the Thalamus in Epilepsy (SANTE) study enrolled 157 patients who met entry criteria similar to the Referral Criteria for general patient selection outlined earlier [3]. Ultimately 110 patients were implanted with bilateral AN DBS electrodes and a single, dual-array pulse generator, and 1 month following surgery, they were randomized to stimulation on or off (sham stimulation). One difficulty with this study was the duration of the subsequent blinded phase, which was only 3 months. At the end of the blinded phase, all patients were crossed-over into an open-label phase, in which all patients received active stimulation for an additional 9 months, to complete the 1-year duration of the primary study. A long-term follow-up then continued to monitor available patients for 2 and 3 years.

The primary end point of the study was the difference between stimulation on and off groups across the blinded phase. There was an improvement of just over 20% in both groups during the 1 month prior to randomization. There was no significant difference between groups in additional change in seizure frequency from the end of the first month through the first 2 months of randomization. During the third month, however, there was a significant difference between groups, with the stimulation on patients having on average a doubling of the post-surgical insertional effect (40.4% improvement), while the stimulation off patients decline to only 14.5% improvement by the end of the sham stimulation period. In the stimulation on group, there was one patient who was noted to have met the criteria of a statistical outlier. This patient also had a fairly unique response to stimulation, with onset of several hundred brief partial seizures soon after turning the stimulation on repeatedly over the first 3 days of stimulation onset. This was a new type of seizure for this patient who did not experience these frequent brief partial seizures before surgery, and they correlated with the stimulation cycling parameters. Stimulation intensity was reduced by 1 V and this resolved the patient's new-onset seizures. This patient ultimately went on to have an excellent long-term result, with a substantial decrease in the frequency of his baseline seizures. Therefore, in addition to meeting statistical outlier criteria, this patient appeared to have essentially a stimulation-related adverse event rather than a true increase in baseline seizures, which as expected for this type of event resolved with cessation of stimulation and eventually alteration in the stimulation parameters. With that single outlier removed, there was a significant difference between on and off groups in the overall treatment effect across the entire 3-month blinded phase of the study. Other statistically significant findings between groups in the blinded phase were seizure-related injuries (7% on versus 26% off), reduction in prospective patient-defined "most severe" seizures (40% on versus 20% off), and a specific reduction in complex-partial seizures (36% on versus 12% off). It is difficult to recommend that AN DBS is most effective for complex partial seizures, since these occurred in over 90% of patients in both groups at baseline, while generalized-from-onset seizures occurred in only 5% of patients in each group prior to surgery.

The results of this study, including the adverse events outlined in detail later, have been presented to regulatory agencies in both the USA and Europe. In Europe, this has led to approval of AN DBS for use in medication-resistant epilepsy, and this device is currently available and being utilized in general epilepsy surgery practice. In the USA, the advisory panel of the FDA which reviewed the data voted to recommend approval, but as of the writing of this chapter, the FDA has failed to approve AN DBS for commercial sale. One ongoing point of contention remains the longevity of the blinded phase of the study, which was a relatively brief 3 months. However, the long-term follow-up results have also been encouraging. In the intent-to-treat group, the 3-month rate of seizure reduction was relatively stable at 1 year (44%), which now included the sham stimulation patients who were crossed-over to stimulation on and thus reduced to the same level as those on stimulation during the blinded phase, and this rate further improved at 2 years (57%). Ongoing study is needed to better define features that may predict optimal outcome, particularly in subsets of patients groups.

Most common programming settings

For most studies of DBS for epilepsy, regardless of target, high-frequency stimulation (at least 100 Hz or greater) has been used. This is based upon the presumption that inhibition of abnormal electrical activity is necessary to halt the spread of seizures and the belief that high-frequency stimulation tends to inhibit neuronal firing and/or drive afferent inhibitory inputs to a given structure. For the SANTE study, which used the Medtronic Kinetra pulse generator, a fixed stimulation paradigm was used for all patients during the blinded phase, with an amplitude of 5 V, pulse width of 90 µs, and frequency of 145 Hz. Changes in voltage up to 7.5 V or frequency up to 185 Hz were permissible during the later half of the open-label phase, and complete freedom for any safe program was permitted once patients completed 1 year and entered the long-term follow-up phase. This is consistent with most of the pilot studies, which also utilized high frequencies and relatively high voltages. One consequence of the high amplitude, which has similarly been seen in DBS for dystonia, is a far greater frequency of IPG changes due to batteries reaching end of life in a shorter time period. The advent of rechargeable IPGs for DBS, which have long been available for spinal cord stimulation, should help to somewhat alleviate this problem. Cycling was also used for these parameters, with stimulation on for 1 min and off for 5 min. This helps to reduce the risk of tissue damage at such high amplitudes and also helps to extend battery life. This again is similar to most pilot studies, although certain earlier studies stimulated at amplitudes of up to 10 V. The stimulation parameters for other targets are a bit more variable because of the nature of small, open-label studies and perhaps the location of the targets. Certain CM DBS studies, for example, have used lower voltages (2–4 V) but far higher pulse widths (300 µs). The earliest CM study by Velasco et al. [10]

actually used lower frequency stimulation (60 Hz) but with a very broad pulse width (1 ms).

Potential side effects and complications

As with all DBS, adverse effects and complications can be divided into two categories: surgical complications and stimulation-related adverse effects. Surgical complications are generally infrequent and most are similar to those observed in more traditional DBS applications for movement disorders. These include infection and hemorrhage, which in the SANTE study occurred in 9.1% and 4.5% of patients respectively. These are similar rates to other major studies of DBS for PD, and none of the hemorrhages in the SANTE study was symptomatic or clinically significant. Another complication of DBS surgery is misplaced leads, which require revision. This rate can vary depending upon the difficulty of the target. Since the AN is a periventricular structure fairly close to midline, it can sometimes be difficult to target and often only one or two contacts will actually be within the nucleus (Figure 8.1). Sometimes large ependymal veins on the ventricular surface of the thalamus can also necessitate unusual trajectories which can further increase the difficulty of placing at least one effective contact within the AN. Finally, many patients being considered for DBS have had prior failed resective surgery or have structural anomalies, either of which can create substantial asymmetry in the brain and particular in the ventricular anatomy. Therefore, unlike movement disorders patients who rarely have had prior brain surgery and whose electrodes target regions that are relatively symmetrical bilaterally,

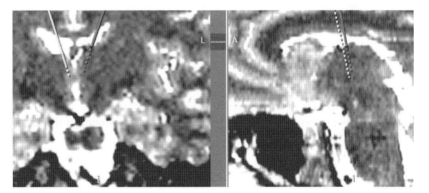

Figure 8.1 Target plan to place bilateral deep brain stimulation electrodes into the anterior nucleus of the thalamus (AN) for a SANTE study patient. Note the asymmetry of the ventricular system on coronal imaging (left). On the sagittal view roughly 6 mm lateral to midline (right), the entry into the anterior nucleus is at the apex of the thalamus just behind the caudate eminence anteriorly. Note the presence of a vein overlying the medial (left) and anterior (right) ependymal surface of the anterior nucleus, requiring a more lateral trajectory to enter the left thalamus.

the AN can exhibit substantial asymmetry that can further complicate targeting. As a result, it is not surprising that another complication in the SANTE study was leads implanted outside of the AN which required replacement. This occurred in 8.2% of patients, which is somewhat higher than the rate of lead revisions due to mistargeting reported in most studies of DBS for movement disorders [3].

Certain stimulation-related adverse effects reflect the local anatomical environment surrounding the electrode. For movement disorders surgery, stimulation of adjacent white matter tracts can lead to paresthesias, motor contractions, speech, or oculomotor difficulties. Paresthesias have also been reported with targets for epilepsy, such as AN. However, given the known function of the circuit of Papez and the role of the AN in learning and memory, it is not entirely surprising that 13% of patients with active stimulation during the blinded phase in the SANTE study reported subjective memory impairments, compared with only 1.8% of sham patients [3]. While this difference was statistically significant, none of these were rated as serious and interestingly there were no deficits or differences between groups on objective neuropsychological testing. Another stimulation-related adverse event was depression, which was also significantly different between active and sham groups, with nearly 15% of stimulated patients demonstrating worsening depression compared with baseline. This resolved over an average of 2–3 months in half of these patients. It is possible that this may reflect stimulation spreading ventrally to the dorsomedial nucleus, which defines the inferior border of the AN and which usually harbors at least one DBS contact in order to effectively anchor the electrode in the brain without slipping back into the ventricle. Adverse events from stimulation at other targets have been less well characterized, because studies have been much smaller and less definitive. Few stimulation-related adverse events have been reported for the CM nucleus, and stimulation of the STN in epilepsy is prone to the same type of adverse events from spread to nearby white matter tracts as described above for movement disorders surgery (Chapter 3).

Conclusions

AN DBS in refractory epilepsy not suitable for resective surgery seems to be safe, reduces seizure frequency, and improves quality of life, but is dependent on patient selection, precise surgical technique, and tailored DBS programming.

References

1 Tellez-Zenteno, J.F., Dhar, R. & Wiebe, S. (2005) Long-term seizure outcomes following epilepsy surgery: a systematic review and meta-analysis. *Brain: A Journal of Neurology*, **128** (Pt 5), 1188–1198.

2 Al-Otaibi, F.A., Hamani, C. & Lozano, A.M. (2011) Neuromodulation in epilepsy. *Neurosurgery*, **69** (4), 957–979; discussion 979.

3 Fisher, R., Salanova, V., Witt T. *et al.* (2010) Electrical stimulation of the anterior nucleus of thalamus for treatment of refractory epilepsy. *Epilepsia*, **51** (5), 899–908.

4 Velasco, F., Velasco, M., Jiménez, F. *et al.* (2000) Predictors in the treatment of difficult-to-control seizures by electrical stimulation of the centromedian thalamic nucleus. *Neurosurgery*, **47** (2), 295–304; discussion 304–305.

5 Hamani, C., Dubiela, F.P., Soares, J.C.K. *et al.* (2010) Anterior thalamus deep brain stimulation at high current impairs memory in rats. *Experimental Neurology*, **225** (1), 154–162.

6 Fisher, R.S., Uematsu, S., Krauss, G.L. *et al.* (1992) Placebo-controlled pilot study of centromedian thalamic stimulation in treatment of intractable seizures. *Epilepsia*, **33** (5), 841–851.

7 Benabid, A.L. Minotti, L., Koudsié, A. *et al.* (2002) Antiepileptic effect of high-frequency stimulation of the subthalamic nucleus (corpus luysi) in a case of medically intractable epilepsy caused by focal dysplasia: a 30-month follow-up: technical case report. *Neurosurgery*, **50** (6), 1385–1391; discussion 1391–1392.

8 Chabardes, S., Kahane, P. & Minotti, L. *et al.* (2002) Deep brain stimulation in epilepsy with particular reference to the subthalamic nucleus. *Epileptic Disorders: International Epilepsy Journal With Videotape*, **4** (Suppl. 3), S83–S93.

9 Cooper, I.S., Upton, A.R. & Amin, I. (1980) Reversibility of chronic neurologic deficits. Some effects of electrical stimulation of the thalamus and internal capsule in man. *Applied Neurophysiology*, **43** (3–5), 244–258.

10 Velasco, F., Velasco, M., Ogarrio, C. & Fanghanel, G. (1987) Electrical stimulation of the centromedian thalamic nucleus in the treatment of convulsive seizures: a preliminary report. *Epilepsia*, **28** (4), 421–430.

Chapter 9

Deep Brain Stimulation in Obsessive Compulsive Disorders

David Christmas[1] and Loes Gabriëls[2]

[1]Ninewells Hospital and Medical School, Dundee, UK
[2]University Hospitals, Leuven, Belgium

Introduction

Since the late 1980s, stimulation of key brain areas has been explored as an alternative to ablative surgery for psychiatric illness, with the first published reports of continuous stimulation emerging in 1999 [1]. It is often suggested that the reversibility of deep brain stimulation (DBS) makes it an attractive alternative to ablative neurosurgery, although the risks arising from implantation of leads and neurostimulators may not be reversible.

The most compelling advantage of DBS is that it allows randomized and double-blinded studies to be conducted. Crossover and staggered-onset research designs permit the differentiation between effects of stimulation, effects of neurosurgery, and the impact of intensified contact with professionals that clinical studies involve.

Rationale of deep brain stimulation in obsessive compulsive disorder

DBS was first used for the treatment of movement disorders where the functional anatomical pathways are well understood. With regards to OCD, there is convergent information pointing to dysfunction within cortico-striatal-thalamic-cortical (CSTC) loops in the pathogenesis of the symptoms.

Neurostimulation: Principles and Practice, First Edition. Edited by Sam Eljamel and Konstantin V. Slavin.

Such pathways may underlie common components in movement disorders and OCD, with overactivation of the 'direct pathway' (cortex to striatum, GPi, thalamus, and back to cortex) contributing to the intrusive and repetitive thoughts and behaviours which characterize OCD.

In particular, some researchers have suggested that a lack of inhibition from the ventromedial (limbic) portions of the striatum may contribute to "aberrant positive feedback loops" in these circuits [2]. It has been argued that the increased metabolism in orbitofrontal regions reflects increases in attempts to control aberrant thoughts [3]. Such speculations are supported by imaging studies which highlight functional abnormalities that normalize with treatment. However, it should be recognized that findings in functional imaging studies of OCD are not unequivocal and the structure and functions of these complex and multiply connected circuits are still being understood.

Deep brain stimulation targets in obsessive compulsive disorders

Current targets have emerged from a variety of mechanisms. DBS of the internal capsule was derived empirically from experience with bilateral anterior capsulotomy. Stimulation of the subthalamic nucleus evolved serendipitously from treatment of patients with Parkinson's disease (PD) who suffered from comorbid OCD. Other targets have developed out of a greater understanding of the neuroanatomical pathways involved in OCD.

Anterior limb of internal capsule and ventral capsule/ventral striatum (VC/VS)

Although the internal capsule was the first target investigated, it was recognized early on that stimulation probably involved the nucleus accumbens [4]. Indeed, subsequent publications have adopted the term ventral capsule/ventral striatum (VC/VS) to reflect the close proximity of these targets.

Nucleus accumbens

Sturm and colleagues [5] first stimulated the right nucleus accumbens (NAcc) as a target in OCD in 2003, based on presumptions about the shell of the NAcc acting as a "bottleneck" for information originating in the amygdala to the basal ganglia, mediodorsal thalamus, and prefrontal cortex.

Inferior thalamic peduncle

Jiménez et al. [6] initially reported two cases (one with OCD and one with major depression) who underwent stimulation of the inferior thalamic peduncle (ITP), and have gone on to describe outcomes for a total of five patients with OCD undergoing ITP stimulation [7]. Benefits are argued to be easy identification of the target through electrophysiological recording.

Subthalamic nucleus

Small case reports of patients with OCD undergoing subthalamic nucleus (STN) DBS for PD reported improvements in symptoms of OCD and the movement disorder [8,9]. Further, the STN appears to play a role in the integration of motor and emotional aspects of behaviour [10], and primate models demonstrate the capacity for STN stimulation to reduce stereotyped behaviour [11].

Patient selection and assessments

Most of the larger centres indicate that DBS for OCD should only be considered for patients (aged 18–60 years) who meet the following conditions:

(1) Primary diagnosis of OCD according to Diagnostic and Statistical Manual of Mental Disoders–IV (or International statistical Classification of Diseases and Related Health Problems–10), based on structured clinical interview.
(2) Yale-Brown Obsessive-Compulsive Scale (Y-BOCS) score ≥30.
(3) Global Assessment of Functioning (GAF) ≤40.
(4) Demonstrated impaired functioning of at least 5 years' duration.
(5) Able to provide informed consent and comply with follow-up requirements.

Most studies require patients to have failed to respond to at least 20 sessions of exposure and response prevention (ERP), but this should be considered a minimum level of behavior therapy.

The complexity, severity, and treatment needs for such patients require well-established multidisciplinary teams of psychiatrists, therapists, and neurosurgeons. Behavioural therapy and family support is required postoperatively. Finally, such patients require long-term commitments to follow-up irrespective of their response to treatment or participation in research studies, and an infrastructure to support this is required.

Evidence level to date

Patients treated with deep brain stimulation for obsessive compulsive disorder: Characteristics

Data have been extracted from 18 published studies and case reports of DBS for OCD. Five reports were single case reports; four reported outcomes for two cases; and the rest included between four and 26 subjects. The largest study ($n = 26$) is a composite report from multiple sites [12].

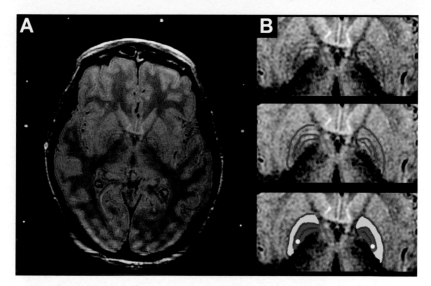

Figure 7.1 Neuroanatomy of the lentiform nucleus and magnetic resonance imaging (MRI) correlates (A) stereotactic axial proton density MRI at the anterior commissure-posterior commissure (AC-PC) level. (See text for full caption.)

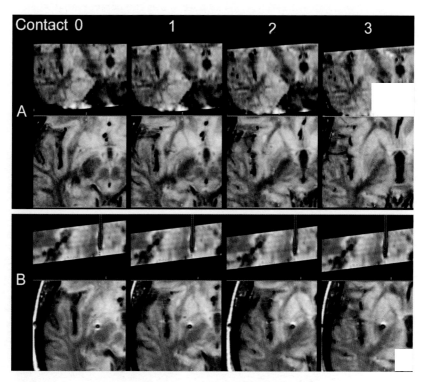

Figure 7.2 Pallidal deep brain stimulation: stereotactic planning and verification of contact location. Stereotactic proton density magnetic resonance images. (See text for full caption.)

Neurostimulation: Principles and Practice, First Edition. Edited by Sam Eljamel and Konstantin V. Slavin.
© 2013 John Wiley & Sons, Ltd. Published 2013 by John Wiley & Sons, Ltd.

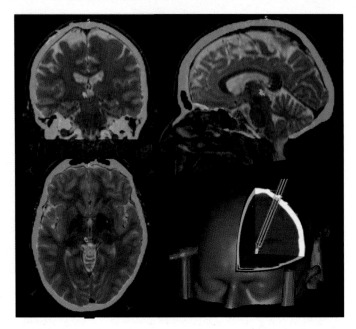

Figure 11.1 Planning a periventricular gray, periacqueduct gray deep brain stimulation trajectory. This figure shows the postoperative computed tomography head scan superimposed on the preoperative magnetic resonance image, using the Medtronic Stealth Station® (Medtronic, Minneapolis). The electrode is clearly visible in the periventricular region and the trajectory of the electrode has been mapped on the 3D image (bottom right).

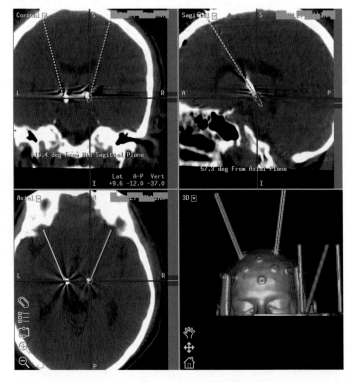

Figure AII.5 Screenshot of fused post DBS implantation CT merged with the preoperative MRI-based targets demonstrating perfect alignment of the plan trajectories and target to the implanted DBS leads.

A total of 105 subjects (59 male; 42 female; four not reported) were identified: USA (*n* = 30); France (*n* = 24); Netherlands (*n* = 17); Germany (*n* = 14); Belgium (*n* = 11); Mexico (*n* = 5); Taiwan (*n* = 4). Targets were VC/VS (*n* = 55; 52.4%); NAcc (*n* = 23; 21.9%); STN (*n* = 22; 21.0%); and ITP (*n* = 5; 4.8%). Data were absent for some subjects.

Mean (±SD) age at surgery (*n* = 101) was 39.1 ± 10.1 (range 21-65) years; mean age at onset of illness (*n* = 100) was 15.1 ± 6.6 (range 4-35) years; and mean duration of illness (*n* = 100) was 23.8 ± 10.2 (range 5-48) years. The mean baseline Y-BOCS, where reported (*n* = 101), was 33.3 ± 3.7 (range 23-40) years. The mean GAF score at baseline (*n* = 57) was 33.0 ± 7.9 (range 10-61 years).

Comorbidities

Comorbid conditions such as depression are common in OCD and probably affect outcome [13]. Axis I comorbidity was reported in 54 out of 105 subjects (51.4%), with the majority of these being major depression (46/105; 43.8%). Many subjects without a formal diagnosis of depression had depression rating scale scores in the "depressed" range, and 75 out of 105 (71.4%) subjects either had a recorded diagnosis of major depression or depression rating scale scores of at least "mild" severity.

In most studies, patients with a history of unstably remitted substance abuse were excluded. However, a number of patients reported by the Mexican team had substance misuse (including cocaine misuse), and investigators should be alert to relationships between substance misuse and OCD [14].

Axis II (Personality) comorbidity is also reported in the literature, although most studies do not report personality assessments. The effects of Axis II comorbidity on outcome from DBS for OCD is unclear, and published studies currently report insufficient information to determine this in individual cases: personality was not reported for approximately 75% of all subjects.

Perioperative and postoperative programming

The use of multipolar leads with four or more individual electrodes per lead allows flexibility in the spatial distribution of the current delivered. However, this flexibility requires extensive testing to maximize benefits and minimize adverse effects. In initial test sessions, both monopolar and bipolar electrode configurations are tested to observe acute stimulation effects. The observations during these sessions usually give an indication of which electrode configurations are used for chronic stimulation. Multiple, often transient, acute effects such as autonomic changes and effects on sensation, motor function, mood, or thinking are seen [15,16].

For chronic stimulation, the choice of the optimal electrode configuration and other stimulation parameters is an iterative process requiring multiple programming visits. Assessments of therapeutic improvement and tolerability are based on patient reports; reports from carers; clinical judgment; and validated rating scales. Especially during the first year of follow-up, patients require close monitoring for deterioration in psychiatric status or stimulation-related adverse effects.

Outcome of deep brain stimulation in obsessive compulsive disorder

The median (range) percentage change on the Y-BOCS for the 58 of 105 (55.2%) patients where pre- and post-DBS Y-BOCS scores reported was 44.0% (0.0–97.4%). The mean (±SD) improvement in GAF score was 31.6 ± 18.9.

Out of 64 subjects where response was defined as ≥35% improvement in Y-BOCS score, 39 (60.9%) were responders. However, it was not possible to determine such an outcome for 39% of subjects. Of 101 subjects for whom it was possible to track across studies (this may include duplicate patients), 64 (63.4%) were reported by the authors as having improved by at least 25%.

Clinical outcomes and symptom domain are reported inconsistently (and not always for individual patients) and it was not possible to determine the predominant symptom cluster for 46 cases (43.8%). However, where both are reported, response rates by main symptom domain, using the categories described by Mataix-Cols *et al.* [17] are contamination/cleaning (*n* = 26), 38.5%; hoarding (*n* = 4), 25.0%; obsessions/checking (*n* = 19), 73.7%; symmetry/ordering (*n* = 10), 50.0%.

In many cases, the very small numbers (and different imaging modalities) mean that caution should be exercised when interpreting imaging findings. However, the reported changes are largely consistent with the current presumptions about the neuroanatomical basis of OCD. For example, chronic stimulation of the VC/VS has been reported to result in modulation of activity in regions such as orbitofrontal cortex, subgenual cingulate, amygdala, and striatum.

Most common programming settings

Optimum parameters have yet to be identified and may not exist. In published studies, stimulation parameters were reported for 62 (59.0%) of subjects, with considerable variability between targets and subjects. For example, amplitude (Volts) ranged from 2.5 to 6.5 V for NAcc DBS (*n* = 18) and from 2.0 to 10.5 for VC/VS (*n* = 37). There was also wide variation in frequency (100–185 Hz) and pulse width (60–450 μs). Importantly, parameters change over time, so published settings may provide an unreliable guide for individual patients.

Potential side effects and complications

Rates of hardware-related adverse effects in psychiatric DBS are similar to those reported in DBS for movement disorders and some technical related issues are likely to be increased where expertise is being developed.

There have been reports of increased risk of suicide with STN stimulation [18], and mood changes (including hypomania) are often reported following DBS for OCD [19,20], particularly with VC/VS and NAcc targets.

Neuropsychological outcomes are partially reported in recent studies, although measures vary and detailed and/or comparable neuropsychological outcomes are infrequent. Based on available data, postoperative neuropsychological impairment appears rare.

Few studies report prospective assessments of personality. This may reflect assumptions that changes in personality are unlikely. However, many studies report effects on mood and anxiety [15,21], libido [22], and stimulation-related disinhibition [4]. Future research should attempt to assess changes in personality, particularly given the potential role that areas such as the ventral striatum may play in personality [23].

Conclusions

DBS for OCD remains in its infancy and although there are increasing numbers of studies reporting outcomes and clinical experiences, large double-blind studies have yet to be performed. Despite this, where conventional treatments are ineffective and the patient remains disabled by symptoms, DBS may offer an alternative to ablative neurosurgery.

References

1 Nuttin, B., Cosyns, P., Demeulemeester, H. et al. (1999) Electrical stimulation in anterior limbs of internal capsules in patients with obsessive-compulsive disorder. Lancet, **354**, 1526.

2 Modell, J.G., Mountz, J.M., Curtis, G.C. et al. (1989) Neurophysiologic dysfunction in basal ganglia/limbic striatal and thalamocortical circuits as a pathogenetic mechanism of obsessive-compulsive disorder. The Journal of Neuropsychiatry and Clinical Neurosciences, **1**, 27-36.

3 Insel, T.R. (1992) Toward a neuroanatomy of obsessive-compulsive disorder. Archives of General Psychiatry, **49**, 739-744.

4 Nuttin, B.J., Gabriëls, L.A., Cosyns, P.R. et al. (2003) Long-term electrical capsular stimulation in patients with obsessive-compulsive disorder. Neurosurgery, **52**, 1263-1274.

5 Sturm, V., Lenartz, D., Koulousakis, A. et al. (2003) The nucleus accumbens: a target for deep brain stimulation in obsessive-compulsive- and anxiety-disorders. Journal of Chemical Neuroanatomy, **26**, 293-299.

6 Jiménez, F., Velasco, F., Salin-Pascual, R. et al. (2007) Neuromodulation of the inferior thalamic peduncle for major depression and obsessive compulsive disorder. Acta Neurochirurgica, **97**, 393-398.

7 Jiménez-Ponce, F., Velasco-Campos, F., Castro-Farfan, G. et al. (2009) Preliminary study in patients with obsessive-compulsive disorder treated with electrical stimulation in the inferior thalamic peduncle. Neurosurgery, **65**, 203-209.

8 Fontaine, D., Mattei, V., Borg, M. *et al.* (2004) Effect of subthalamic nucleus stimulation on obsessive-compulsive disorder in a patient with Parkinson disease. Case report. *Journal of Neurosurgery*, **100**, 1084-1086.

9 Mallet, L., Mesnage, V., Houeto, J.L. *et al.* (2002) Compulsions, Parkinson's disease, and stimulation. *Lancet*, **360**, 1302-1304.

10 Mallet, L., Schüpbach, M., N'Diaye, K. *et al.* (2007) Stimulation of subterritories of the subthalamic nucleus reveals its role in the integration of the emotional and motor aspects of behavior. *Proceedings of the National Academy of Sciences of the United States of America*, **104**, 10661-10666.

11 Baup, N., Grabli, D., Karachi, C. *et al.* (2008) High-frequency stimulation of the anterior subthalamic nucleus reduces stereotyped behaviors in primates. *Journal of Neuroscience*, **28**, 8785-8788.

12 Greenberg, B.D., Gabriels, L.A., Malone, D.A., Jr *et al.* (2010) Deep brain stimulation of the ventral internal capsule/ventral striatum for obsessive-compulsive disorder: worldwide experience. *Molecular Psychiatry*, **15**, 64-79.

13 Overbeek, T., Schruers, K., Vermetten, E. *et al.* (2002) Comorbidity of obsessive-compulsive disorder and depression: prevalence, symptom severity, and treatment effect. *Journal of Clinical Psychology*, **63**, 1106-1112.

14 Crum, R.M. & Anthony, J.C. (1993) Cocaine use and other suspected risk factors for obsessive-compulsive disorder: a prospective study with data from the Epidemiologic Catchment Area surveys. *Drug and Alcohol Dependence*, **31**, 281-295.

15 Greenberg, B.D., Malone, D.A., Friehs, G.M. *et al.* (2006) Three-year outcomes in deep brain stimulation for highly resistant obsessive-compulsive disorder. *Neuropsychopharm*, **31**, 2384-2393.

16 Gabriëls, L., Kuyck, K.V., Welkenhuyzen, M. *et al.* (2008) Deep brain stimulation in obsessive-compulsive disorder. In: D. Tarsy, J.L. Vitek, P. Starr & M.S. Okun (eds), *Current Clinical Neurology: Deep Brain Stimulation in Neurological and Psychiatric Disorders*, pp. 531-546. Humana Press, Totowa, NJ.

17 Mataix-Cols, D., do Rosario-Campos, M.C. & Leckman, J.F. (2005) A multidimensional model of obsessive-compulsive disorder. *The American Journal of Psychiatry*, **162**, 228-238.

18 Rodrigues, A.M., Rosas, M.J., Gago, M.F. *et al.* (2010) Suicide attempts after subthalamic nucleus stimulation for Parkinson's disease. *European Neurology*, **63**, 176-179.

19 Huff, W., Lenartz, D., Schormann, M. *et al.* (2010) Unilateral deep brain stimulation of the nucleus accumbens in patients with treatment-resistant obsessive-compulsive disorder: outcomes after one year. *Clinical Neurology and Neurosurgery*, **112**, 137-143.

20 Mantione, M., van de Brink, W., Schuurman, P.R. *et al.* (2010) Smoking cessation and weight loss after chronic deep brain stimulation of the nucleus accumbens: therapeutic and research implications: case report. *Neurosurgery*, **66**, E218.

21 Mallet, L., Polosan, M., Jaafari, N. *et al.* (2008) Subthalamic nucleus stimulation in severe obsessive-compulsive disorder. *The New England Journal of Medicine*, **359**, 2121-2134.

22 Denys, D., Mantione, M., Figee, M. *et al.* (2010) Deep brain stimulation of the nucleus accumbens for treatment-refractory obsessive-compulsive disorder. *Archives of General Psychiatry*, **67**, 1061-1068.

23 Cohen, M.X., Schoene-Bake, J.-C., Elger, C.E. *et al.* (2009) Connectivity-based segregation of the human striatum predicts personality characteristics. *Nature Neuroscience*, **12**, 32-34.

Chapter 10

Deep Brain Stimulation in Treatment of Refractory Major Depression

Clement Hamani[1] and Paul E. Holtzheimer[2]

[1]Toronto Western Hospital and Centre for Addiction and Mental Health, Toronto, Ontario, Canada

[2]Geisel School of Medicine at Dartmouth, Dartmouth Hitchcock Medical Center, Lebanon, New Hampshire, USA

Introduction

Depression is a common psychiatric disorder with a 6 months' prevalence of approximately 5% [1]. In the USA alone, around 20 million people have been diagnosed with this disorder, which is associated with an important socioeconomic burden [2].

The initial therapeutic approach for patients with depression consists of medications and/or psychotherapy with a positive response (typically defined as a 50% decrease in severity from baseline) on the order of 60-70%. However, full remission is less common and relapse rates are high. Patients who do not present a favorable outcome with these treatments are considered to have chronic and refractory forms of the disorder [3,4]. Therapeutic alternatives for this population include the use of different classes of medications, including a number of augmentation strategies, and electroconvulsive therapy (ECT). In patients who are still unresponsive, surgical interventions have been proposed.

Until recently, stereotactic lesions were considered the surgical treatment of choice. Over the last 15 years, however, invasive neuromodulation strategies have been investigated. The appeal of these techniques is that stimulation induced side effects may be reversed and titrated by changing stimulation settings or turning off the DBS system. Invasive neuromodulation therapies

Neurostimulation: Principles and Practice, First Edition. Edited by Sam Eljamel and Konstantin V. Slavin.

studied to date include vagus nerve stimulation (VNS), cortical stimulation, and deep brain stimulation (DBS). All require surgical intervention for the implantation of electrodes, either wrapped around the vagus nerve, directly on the surface of the dura mater/cerebral cortex, or deep into the brain parenchyma (DBS).

In this chapter, we review the clinical outcome of DBS in various targets for the treatment of refractory major depression (TRMD).

Diagnostic criteria in major depression disorder

According to the Diagnostic and Statistical Manual of Mental Disorders 4th Edition (DMS-IV), diagnostic criteria for major depression disorder (MDD) involve the presence of single or multiple major depressive episodes (MDEs), as well as the absence of manic, mixed (combined depressive and manic episode), or hypomanic episodes. Bipolar I disorder involves a combination of both MDEs and manic, hypomanic and/or mixed episodes. Bipolar II is characterized by the presence of MDEs and hypomanic episodes.

For the diagnosis of a MDE, patients must present at least five of the following symptoms for at least 2 weeks: depressed mood, markedly diminished interest or pleasure and/or significant apathy, significant change in appetite or weight, insomnia or hypersomnia, psychomotor agitation or retardation, fatigue or loss of energy, a feeling of worthlessness, excessive or inappropriate guilt, or loss of self-esteem, indecisiveness or diminished ability to think or concentrate, recurrent thoughts of death or suicidal ideas without a specific plan, a specific plan for suicide, or an actual attempt. At least one of the five symptoms necessary to diagnose an MDE must be a loss of interest or pleasure or depressed mood that persists during most of the day, nearly every day. In addition to these criteria, symptoms must not be secondary to substance abuse or medication use, underlying medical conditions, or to bereavement. They must represent a change from antecedent functioning and cause marked distress or significant impairment of social or occupational functioning.

Deep brain stimulation

As previously mentioned, DBS entails the delivery of electrical current into the brain parenchyma through implanted electrodes. DBS surgery involves the implantation of an electrode into a specific target, selected based on imaging studies (i.e., magnetic resonance imaging, computed tomography). Microelectrode mapping of the target is used in many centers to record the physiological activity of local neuronal population and distinguish borders between grey and white matter. Once implanted, the DBS electrode is connected to an implantable pulse generator (IPG), usually placed in the infra-clavicular region, through extension cables. Electrodes in currently available commercial systems have four contacts through which current may be delivered. Settings that can be modulated include the stimulation amplitude (volts or milliamps), pulse width (microseconds) and frequency (Hertz). In addition, one may choose contacts to be used as cathodes and anodes (the IPG may also be chosen as the anode).

DBS targets proposed to date for the surgical treatment of depression are the subcallosal cingulate gyrus (SCG), the inferior thalamic peduncle (ITP), the nucleus accumbens (Acb), the VC/VS, and lateral habenula (LHb).

Surgical candidates

Though some variability exists in the inclusion criteria to select patients for DBS, most studies reviewed in this chapter have some features in common. Overall, patients had to fulfill diagnostic criteria for major depressive disorder or bipolar II, with the last major depressive episode persisting for over 1 year. Severity of disease had to be recorded with validated scales such as the Hamilton Depression Scale (HAMD), Montgomery–Asberg Depression Scale (MADRS), and Global Assessment of Function scores. Patients must have failed multiple treatments, including different antidepressant medications, psychotherapy, and often ECT. In addition, most trials excluded patients with overt manic features, imminent suicidal plans, other major Axis I or II disorders, and neurological or clinical conditions that could interfere with the surgical procedure.

In most trials, response to treatment was defined as a ≥50% improvement in selected depression scales (i.e., HAMD, MADRS), and remission was based on an absolute cut-off on the rating scale chosen.

The rationale for deep brain stimulation in treatment of refractory major depression

Subcallosal cingulate gyrus

The rationale for targeting the SCG stems largely from imaging work [5]. Cerebral blood flow and metabolic activity increases in this region when healthy subjects are asked to rehearse autobiographic sad scripts and when previously depressed subjects undergo tryptophan depletion (i.e., ultimately leading to a reduction in serotonin brain levels) (for a review see Agid et al. [6]). Further, some patients with severe depression have an overall increase in baseline SCG metabolic activity [7]. After treatment with various antidepressants, transcranial magnetic stimulation, or ECT, this pattern is reversed with a reduction in SCG metabolism. Based on these findings, initial DBS trials proposed that the delivery of stimulation to the SCG could disrupt abnormal activity in the neurocircuitry of depression.

A few groups have published their results on SCG DBS for depression (Figure 10.1). Overall, 30–65% of patients have been considered to be responders at

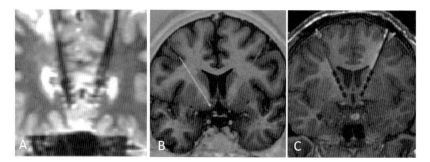

Figure 10.1 Coronal sections of imaging studies showing the location of electrodes contacts or the planned trajectory for electrode implantation in patients treated with subgenual cingulate gyrus (A), nucleus accumbens (B) or ventral capsule/ventral striatum (C) deep brain stimulation. A, Reproduced from [5] with permission from Elsevier; B, reproduced from [18] with permission from Macmillan Publishers Ltd; C, reproduced from [25] with permission from Elsevier.

1 year [7–10]. In the two studies reporting clinical data at longer follow-ups, the percentage of responders was 96% (2 years) [9] and 75% (3 years) [8]. Of note, outcome in patients with major depressive disorder does not seem to differ from that of bipolar II patients [9]. Common stimulation parameters used during programming were 4–8 V/mA, 60–90 μs and 130 Hz.

Though two suicides have been reported with the use of SCG DBS, it is unclear whether these were related to the use of stimulation [8]. The remainder of the side effects were mainly related to the surgical procedure or hardware implants (e.g., hardware infections, pain in the site of the IPG, etc.) [5,7] and were similar to those with DBS in other targets [11]. Neuropsychological assessment 12 months after stimulation onset did not reveal any adverse effects [12].

As the use of DBS is at early stages, biomarkers that may predict who will respond to surgery are still lacking. Imaging studies are being conducted to assess whether morphologic or functional circuitry distinctions can explain why some patients improve with the surgery. Differences in outcome across individuals may not be explained by differences in the location of the electrodes [13]. A recent electrophysiological study has shown that lower theta concordance (a measure of relative and absolute theta rhythms) in frontal regions at baseline and an early increase in this same measure at 1 month predicts a good clinical response [14].

Positron emission tomography (PET) imaging at baseline revealed that patients with depression had an increased metabolism in the SCG and a decreased activity in prefrontal and premotor cortices, the dorsal anterior cingulate gyrus and anterior insula have been reported compared with non-depressed control subjects. Postoperative studies revealed this pattern was reversed in patients who improved with DBS [5,7].

Inforior thalamic peduncle

The ITP comprises a fiber bundle that conveys projections from intralaminar and midline thalamic nuclei to the orbitofrontal cortex [15,16,17]. So far, only one patient with TRMD treated with ITP DBS has been reported in the literature [15]. The patient experienced a significant improvement in her symptoms after the insertion of the electrodes into the target in the absence of stimulation (i.e., insertional effect) with HAMD scores going from 42 (baseline) to 3. At the end of the first postoperative week, the DBS system was activated at 2.5 V, 450 µs, and 130 Hz. During 8 months of continuous stimulation the patient experienced a significant improvement. Double-blinded assessment was then initiated with stimulation being discontinued for 12 months. This culminated in a significant fluctuation of HAMD scores and a deterioration of Global Assessment of Function scores. The benefits of DBS were recaptured when stimulation was reinitiated.

Nucleus accumbens

The rationale for DBS in the Acb involved its position as a relay between limbic and motor circuits as well as the importance of the Acb in mechanisms of reward and motivation, which are disrupted in depressed patients [18].

In a preliminary report, three patients with depression treated with Acb DBS had a significant improvement in anhedonia [18] (Figure 10.1). Based on these results, a series of patients were operated and followed for 1 year. Overall, approximately 45% of subjects were considered to be responders [19]. A subsequent study from the same group has shown that patients who did well at 1 year continue to benefit from the procedure at longer follow-ups (4 years) [20]. Common stimulation parameters in these trials were 130 Hz, 90 µs, and 4–8 V [19,20]. In the group of subjects that did not respond to surgery, one patient committed and another attempted suicide. Additional side effects were similar to those described in other applications of DBS. PET imaging 6 months after stimulation onset has shown a decrease in activity in various prefrontal structures, including the SCG, orbitofrontal cortex, caudate nucleus, and thalamus compared with baseline [19].

Ventral capsule/ventral striatum

The rationale for stimulating the VC/VS to treat depression was based on the improvements in mood observed in patients with OCD treated with DBS in this same target [21,22,23]. Further, stereotactic lesions of the anterior capsule (capsulotomy) have been used to treat psychiatric disorders for many decades.

In an initial open-label trial, 15 patients with refractory depression were treated with VS/VC DBS in three different centers [24] (Figure 10.1). Overall, 40% were considered to be responders at 6 months and 53.3% during the last follow-up. Mean stimulation settings in this group of patients were 7 V,

123 μs, 127 Hz [24]. Side effects were similar to those in other indications of the therapy, except for a somewhat higher incidence of hypomanic episodes, disinhibition, and impulsivity (particularly noted in a patient with bipolar disorder). No neuropsychological changes were noticed after stimulation.

In addition to open-label reports, results of a multicenter, prospective, randomized trial have been reported in meetings [25]. Thirty patients with chronic treatment resistant were implanted with VS/VC electrodes. Active ($n = 15$) or sham stimulation ($n = 14$) was delivered during a 4-month double-blind phase. Twenty percent of the subjects receiving active stimulation and 14.3% in the sham-treated group responded to the surgery. At 1 year, 21% were considered to be responders [25]. Though these results were somewhat disappointing, they point to the clear need for a placebo arm in pivotal clinical trials.

Lateral habenula

The LHb has been targeted in a single patient based on the fact that it receives important serotoninergic, noradrenergic, and dopaminergic innervation, plays a role in the circuitry of reward and is an important structure in animal models of depression and anxiety [26]. In addition, activity in the LHb covaries with that in the dorsal raphe in humans undergoing tryptophan depletion [27]. The patient selected for surgery had a significant improvement with DBS. Switching off the device precipitated a new relapse, which was controlled upon reinstating stimulation [26].

Conclusions

DBS in various brain targets has been investigated as a surgical procedure for the treatment of depression. Overall, in most open-label articles published to date approximately 50% of patients presented a 50% or higher improvement in depressive scores. One of the most important aspects of this field is that we still do not know which patients will respond well to which surgery. Finding biomarkers or clinical features that might forecast a good outcome is imperative. Several groups are now engaged in imaging, electrophysiological, and genetic studies to find predictors of a clinical response and to try to characterize clinical phenotypes that are more responsive to DBS (e.g., melancholic versus non-melancholic patients). An example of a clear predictor of response in functional neurosurgery is the use of the levodopa challenge test in patients with Parkinson's disease treated with STN DBS. Patients undergoing this test are evaluated at baseline (without medication) and after receiving levodopa. The response obtained with this drug gives a general idea about the improvement that might be expected with surgery.

Another important aspect will be to confirm the results of open-label trials with double-blinded studies including sham and active stimulation arms.

Though it has been suggested that the severity of patients included in current trials and the longevity of a DBS response would reduce the chances of a placebo response, recent results of the VS/VC study presented above have proven that this is not necessarily the case.

References

1 Depression Guideline Panel (ed.) (1993) *Depression in primary care: Volume 1 Detection and Diagnosis.* (Clinical Guideline No. 5, AHCPR Publication No. 93-0550). Department of Health and Human Services, Public Health Service, Agency for Health Care Policy and Research.: Rockville, MD: US.

2 Greenberg, P.E., Stiglin, L.E., Finkelstein, S.N. & Berndt, E.R. (1993) The economic burden of depression in 1990. *The Journal of Clinical Psychiatry*, **54**, 405-418.

3 Depression Guideline Panel (ed.) (1993) *Depression in primary care: Volume 2 Treatment of major depression.* (Clinical Guideline No. 5, AHCPR Publication No. 93-0551). Department of Health and Human Services, Public Health Service, Agency for Health Care Policy and Research.: Rockville, MD: US.

4 Guze, S.B. & Robins, E. (1970) Suicide and primary affective disorders. *The British Journal of Psychiatry: The Journal of Mental Science*, **117**, 437-438.

5 Mayberg, H.S., Lozano, A.M., Voon, V. et al. (2005) Deep brain stimulation for treatment-resistant depression. *Neuron*, **45**, 651-660.

6 Agid, Y., Buzsaki, G., Diamond, D.M. et al. (2007) How can drug discovery for psychiatric disorders be improved? *Nature Reviews Drug Discovery*, **6**, 189-201.

7 Lozano, A.M., Mayberg, H.S., Giacobbe, P. et al. (2008) Subcallosal cingulate gyrus deep brain stimulation for treatment-resistant depression. *Biological Psychiatry*, **64**, 461-467.

8 Kennedy, S.H., Giacobbe, P., Rizvi, S.J. et al. (2011) Deep brain stimulation for treatment-resistant depression: follow-up after 3 to 6 years. *The American Journal of Psychiatry*, **168**, 502-510.

9 Holtzheimer, P.E., Kelley, M.E., Gross, R.E. et al. (2012) Subcallosal cingulate deep brain stimulation for treatment-resistant unipolar and bipolar depression. *Archives of General Psychiatry*, **69**, 150-158.

10 Puigdemont, D., Perez-Egea, R., Portella, M.J. et al. (2011) Deep brain stimulation of the subcallosal cingulate gyrus: further evidence in treatment-resistant major depression. *The International Journal of Neuropsychopharmacology*, **22**, 1-13.

11 Hamani, C. & Lozano, A.M. (2006) Hardware-related complications of deep brain stimulation: a review of the published literature. *Stereotactic and Functional Neurosurgery*, **84**, 248-251.

12 McNeely, H.E., Mayberg, H.S., Lozano, A.M. & Kennedy, S.H. (2008) Neuropsychological impact of Cg25 deep brain stimulation for treatment-resistant depression: preliminary results over 12 months. *The Journal of Nervous and Mental Disease*, **196**, 405-410.

13 Hamani, C., Mayberg, H., Snyder, B. et al. (2009) Deep brain stimulation of the subcallosal cingulate gyrus for depression: anatomical location of active contacts in clinical responders and a suggested guideline for targeting. *Journal of Neurosurgery*, **111**, 1209-1215.

14 Broadway, J.M., Holtzheimer, P.E., Hilimire, M.R. *et al.* (2012) Frontal theta cordance predicts 6-month antidepressant response to subcallosal cingulate deep brain stimulation for treatment-resistant depression: a pilot study. *Neuropsychopharmacology*, **37**, 1764-1772.

15 Jimenez, F., Velasco, F., Salin-Pascual, R. *et al.* (2005) A patient with a resistant major depression disorder treated with deep brain stimulation in the inferior thalamic peduncle. *Neurosurgery*, **57**, 585-593; discussion 585-593.

16 Jimenez, F., Velasco, F., Salin-Pascual, R. *et al.* (2007) Neuromodulation of the inferior thalamic peduncle for major depression and obsessive compulsive disorder. *Acta Neurochirurgica. Supplement*, **97**, 393-398.

17 Velasco, F., Velasco, M., Jimenez, F., Velasco, A.L. & Salin-Pascual, R. (2005) Neurobiological background for performing surgical intervention in the inferior thalamic peduncle for treatment of major depression disorders. *Neurosurgery*, **57**, 439-448; discussion 439-448.

18 Schlaepfer, T.E., Cohen, M.X., Frick, C. *et al.* (2008) Deep brain stimulation to reward circuitry alleviates anhedonia in refractory major depression. *Neuropsychopharmacology*, **33**, 368-377.

19 Bewernick, B.H., Hurlemann, R., Matusch, A. *et al.* (2010) Nucleus accumbens deep brain stimulation decreases ratings of depression and anxiety in treatment-resistant depression. *Biological Psychiatry*, **67**, 110-116.

20 Bewernick, B.H., Kayser, S., Sturm, V. & Schlaepfer, T.E. (2012) Long-term effects of nucleus accumbens deep brain stimulation in treatment-resistant depression: evidence for sustained efficacy. *Neuropsychopharmacology*, **37**, 1975-1985.

21 Greenberg, B.D., Malone, D.A., Friehs, G.M. *et al.* (2006) Three-year outcomes in deep brain stimulation for highly resistant obsessive-compulsive disorder. *Neuropsychopharmacology*, **31**, 2384-2393.

22 Nuttin, B., Cosyns, P., Demeulemeester, H., Gybels, J. & Meyerson, B. (1999) Electrical stimulation in anterior limbs of internal capsules in patients with obsessive-compulsive disorder. *Lancet*, **354**, 1526.

23 Nuttin, B.J., Gabriels, L.A., Cosyns, P.R. *et al.* (2003) Long-term electrical capsular stimulation in patients with obsessive-compulsive disorder. *Neurosurgery*, **52**, 1263-1272; discussion 1272-1274.

24 Malone, D.A., Jr, Dougherty, D.D., Rezai, A.R. *et al.* (2009) Deep brain stimulation of the ventral capsule/ventral striatum for treatment-resistant depression. *Biological Psychiatry*, **65**, 267-275.

25 Dougherty, D.D., Carpenter, L.L., Bhati, M.T. *et al.* (2012) A randomized sham-controlled trial of DBS of the VC/VS for treatment-resistant depression. In *67th Annual Scientific Convention and Meeting of the Society-of-Biological-Psychiatry*. Philadelphia.

26 Sartorius, A., Kiening, K.L., Kirsch, P. *et al.* (2010) Remission of major depression under deep brain stimulation of the lateral habenula in a therapy-refractory patient. *Biological Psychiatry*, **67**, e9-e11.

27 Morris, J.S., Smith, K.A., Cowen, P.J. *et al.* (1999) Covariation of activity in habenula and dorsal raphe nuclei following tryptophan depletion. *Neuroimage*, **10**, 163-172.

Chapter 11

Deep Brain Stimulation in Pain Syndromes

Alexander Green

John Radcliffe Hospital, Oxford, UK

Introduction

Neuropathic pain is pain due to damage to the nervous system. In a cross-sectional Canadian sample, 35% reported chronic pain, of which neuro-pathic pain accounted for over half (a prevalence of 17.9%), and 3% reported pain refractory to contemporaneous drug treatment [1]. In one study of 914 patients with limb amputations, almost 80% reported some degree of chronic "phantom" pain, and approximately one-quarter regarded this pain as unac-ceptable, despite maximal drug therapy [2]. Similar figures exist for brachial plexus injury where the nerves to the arm are damaged [3], and both of these patient populations are generally young and of working age (mean age of 50.3 years in the former study and an age range of 16-44 years in the latter study with both studies showing a predominance of males). Living with chronic pain which does not respond to drug therapy is a devastating experi-ence and leads to reduced quality of life and social functioning [4]. Therefore, successful treatment of these patients has significant implications for quality of life, and may lead to a reduction in medications that are likely to be life-long, expensive, and associated with unwanted side effects.

Although deep brain stimulation (DBS) has become well known as an important therapy for treating movement disorders such as Parkinson's disease (PD), tremor, and dystonia, it was in fact used for chronic pain over 50 years ago by stimulating the hypothalamus [5]. Around the same time, lesioning of thalamic nuclei and adjacent structures was used for the allevia-tion of pain [6]. This evidence led investigators to try stimulation of the "sensory thalamus" for treating chronic neuropathic pain [7]. Following this, a variety of brain targets were stimulated.

Neurostimulation: Principles and Practice, First Edition. Edited by Sam Eljamel and Konstantin V. Slavin.

During the past 20 years or so, DBS for pain has only been practiced by a small number of centers worldwide, but success has been reported in many etiologies of neuropathic pain including central post-stroke pain (CPSP), brachial plexus injury, phantom limb pain, spinal pain, and atypical facial pain [8].

Referral criteria

Patients with chronic neuropathic pain are often complex and pain can be very difficult to assess objectively. It is therefore almost mandatory that these patients have been assessed and treated by either a pain physician or a neurologist specializing in chronic pain, before they are referred for DBS. Patients that are suitable for DBS are ones that have pain refractory to multiple medication regimes and multiple classes of analgesics. These include (but are not limited to) antiepileptics such as carbamazepine and gabapentin, opiates including tramadol and morphine, and other classes of drugs such as antidepressants (e.g. tricyclics).

In theory, any patient with a chronic neuropathic pain syndrome may be suitable but the most "successful" indications include phantom limb pain, CPSP, atypical facial pain, anesthesia dolorosa, brachial plexus injury, and spinal pain. Patients should be aware that having a DBS implant will require fairly regular follow-up for programming and battery changes every few years. They should also be aware that DBS rarely removes the pain completely and the intention is to significantly reduce the intensity of the pain. DBS may be contraindicated if there is an increased surgical risk or if the patient has significant comorbidities. Anticoagulation is a relative contraindication.

Rationale of deep brain stimulation for pain

The principle is to insert stimulating electrodes into areas of the brain that are part of the "pain network" and include areas such as the "periaqueductal grey area" (PAG) in the midbrain as well as the "sensory thalamus" (Figure 11.1).

These deep brain areas alter pain in different ways. The PAG is thought to be important for the "descending modulation" of pain, and stimulation of this area (when successful) leads to a replacement of the pain with a feeling of warmth in the affected area. The sensory thalamus is part of a relay station where painful sensations are projected to the cortex and stimulation of this area probably "masks" the pain by providing a "pins and needles" effect, akin to an internal "TENS" machine (a TENS or transcutaneous electrical nerve stimulation device is applied to the skin of a painful area and is similar to rubbing the painful area). Exactly how DBS works is a mystery, but when it works well the procedure can provide profound pain relief in a patient whose pain is refractory to all medication types. Other areas such as the "cingulate cortex" are also being evaluated and, when successful, provide a dissociation between the feeling of pain and its experience − in other words,

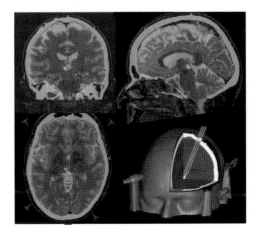

Figure 11.1 Planning a periventricular gray, periaqueduct gray deep brain stimulation trajectory. This figure shows the postoperative computed tomography head scan superimposed on the preoperative magnetic resonance image, using the Medtronic Stealth Station® (Medtronic, Minneapolis). The electrode is clearly visible in the periventricular region and the trajectory of the electrode has been mapped on the 3D image (bottom right). Refer to color plate section for color version of this figure.

the recipient's can feel the pain but it doesn't bother them anymore. In patients with cluster headache, the posterior hypothalamus is stimulated and this target is based on PET studies that showed this area to be overactive during an attack [9].

Assessment methods

Unlike DBS for PD, there are no "standard" methods of assessment of DBS for pain. However, assessments should include some sort of pain scoring system, quality of life measures, and a neuropsychology assessment. The first assessment is made at the time of initially seeing the patient with a frank discussion regarding what DBS may achieve at best and worst, and how the patient may react if there is no effect (which occurs in 20%). An assessment of medical history and discussion of risks should also be done at this time. If the decision is made to go ahead with surgery (either now or after a period to contemplate the issues), the following assessments are made.

(1) Formal neuropsychology tests including memory and attentional batteries but with an emphasis on the pain syndrome and discussions regarding the psychological effects of the pain, an assessment as to whether the pain is exacerbated by psychological factors (that may be treated separately), risks, and expectations of surgery.

(2) Pain scores. These may include
(a) Visual analogue score (twice daily and repeated for 14 days)
(b) A neuropathic pain score such as the McGill Pain Questionnaire or Neuropathic Pain Symptom Inventory
(3) Quality of life/health status
(a) Short Form 36 (SF-36)
(b) EuroQol 5D
(4) Preoperative MRI scan to check no contraindications and for planning if non-MRI compatible frame is being used.

After these assessments are complete, a decision can be made as to whether to proceed with surgery.

Evidence of efficacy

Two multicenter trials of DBS for chronic pain have been conducted by Medtronic Corp. The first trial in 1976 had 196 patients (using the Medtronic Model 3380® electrode) and a second trial in 1990 had 50 patients (using Model 3387®).The two trials were far from ideal as they consisted of case series from various neurosurgical centers, which were not randomized or case controlled, and in addition had poor enrolment and high attrition. Heterogeneous case mixes with unspecified patient selection criteria, and subjective and unblinded assessment of patient outcomes added to the confusion. The study criterion for efficacy was that at least half of patients should report at least 50% pain relief 1 year after surgery. This was not met by either trial, and FDA approval for analgesic DBS was therefore not sought by the device manufacturer. Despite these initial disappointments, pain relief in those who were followed up reached approximately 60% in one of the trials.

As well as the unsuccessful trials, there have been a number of case series of DBS for pain (Table 11.1). Some of these studies report impressive out-

Table 11.1 Summary of case series of deep brain stimulation for pain [10-20]

Author (year)	Number of patients implanted	Number successful initially (%)	Number successful long-term (%)	Follow-up time (months)
Richardson & Akil (1977)	30	27 (90)	18 (60)	1-46
Plotkin (1980)	10	N/A	4 (40)	36
Shulman et al. (1982)	24	18 (67)	11 (46)	>24
Young et al. (1985)	48	43 (89)	35 (73)	2-60
Hosobuchi (1986)	122	105 (86)	94 (77)	24-168
Levy et al. (1987)	141	83 (59)	42 (12)	24-168
Siegfried (1987)	89	N/A	38 (43)	<24
Gybels et al. (1993)	36	22 (61)	11 (31)	48
Kumar et al. (1997)	68	53 (78)	42 (62)	6-180
Owen et al. (2005)	15	12 (80)	9 (60)	48
Hamani et al. (2006)	21	13 (62)	5 (24)	2-108

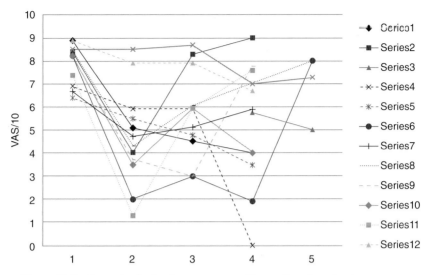

Figure 11.2 Some typical pain scores over time, after deep brain stimulation. This shows both the variability in response but also that some patients become "tolerant" to stimulation over time (Aziz TZ, Green AL, unpublished). VAS, visual analogue scale.

comes with up to 90% initial "success" and up to 77% long-term "success." However, as the reader will see, there are huge variations in "success." At least some of this variation is due to the different etiologies and measurement methods used, but also the varied definitions of "success" between different case series.

Long-term success is also very variable. Figure 11.2 shows a typical group of patients where it can be seen that while some patients retain analgesia, others display a degree of "tolerance" to DBS. These data illustrate two of the fundamental difficulties with this therapy: variation/unpredictability of response to DBS and long-term efficacy. More work is needed to try and solve these problems, for example by using biomarkers to predict individual efficacy and strategies to reduce tolerance. Regarding the lack of randomized controlled trials (RCTs), while RCT evidence may be helpful to predict likelihood of success, as DBS for pain is a "last resort treatment," the benefit of a large RCT is questionable as the real issue for the individual is "are the risks of DBS worth it for the likelihood of success." Most patients are so desperate that they are prepared to take a 0.5% risk of stroke for even a 10% chance it will work!

Most common stimulator settings

Unlike DBS for movement disorders, which generally uses "high"-frequency stimulation (130–180 Hz), in DBS for pain "low" settings are used. These can be anywhere from 5 to 80 Hz, but typical values are between 30 and 50 Hz.

In general, 100 Hz or above can cause pain. Programming is usually a "trial and error" process with a wide range of frequencies tried at different voltages and pulse widths. The contacts used are those that, when stimulated, give sensation in the affected area and can either be bipolar or monopolar. Voltages and pulse widths are then titrated at different frequencies until the best response is achieved. Typical voltages are from 1 to 4 V and pulse widths tend to be higher than in movement disorders with widths of 350 μs not being unusual.

Potential side effects and complications

Complications are those related to the DBS surgery and side effects of stimulation (which are reversible). The risks of DBS for pain are similar to DBS for any condition and include death (0.5%), stroke (1-2%), seizures (2%), infection (5-10%), lead fracture and disconnection (5-10%), and loss of efficacy (see earlier). However, very few of these complications have been reported in case series of DBS for pain.

Stimulation related side-effects include unwanted sensory side effects (burning or intense tingling), gaze and eye movement problems (related to stimulation of the superior colliculus with PAG stimulation), fear and anxiety (PAG). However, these side effects can generally be mitigated by adjustment of the stimulation parameters.

Further reading

Bennett, M. (2011) *Neuropathic Pain (Oxford Pain Management Library Series)*. Oxford University Press, New York, USA.

Cruccua, G., Aziz, T.Z., Garcia-Larrea, L. *et al.* (2007) EFNS guidelines on neurostimulation therapy for neuropathic pain. *European Journal of Neurology*, **14**, 952-970.

Deer, T.R. (2010) *Atlas of Implantable Therapies for Pain Management*. Springer Science+Business Media, New York.

Owen, S.L., Green, A.L., Nandi, D.D. *et al.* (2007) Deep brain stimulation for neuropathic pain. In: D.E. Sakas & B.A. Simpson (eds), *Operative Neuromodulation*, Vol. 2, Neural Networks Surgery, pp. 111-116. SpringerWien, New York.

Pereira, E.A., Moir, L., Green, A.L. & Aziz, T.Z. (2009) Deep brain stimulation for pain. In: E.S. Krames, P.H. Peckham & A.R. Rezai (eds), *Neuromodulation*, pp. 499-507. Academic Press, New York.

References

1 Toth, C., Lander, J. & Wiebe, S. (2009) The prevalence and impact of chronic pain with neuropathic pain symptoms in the general population. *Pain Medicine*, **10** (5), 918-929.

2 Ephraim, P.L., Wegener, S.T., MacKenzie, E.J. *et al.* (2005) Phantom pain, residual limb pain, and back pain In amputees. results of a national survey. *Archives of Physical Medicine and Rehabilitation,* **86** (10), 1910-1919.

3 Waikakul, S., Waikakul, W. & Pausawasdi, S. (2000) Brachial plexus injury and pain: incidence and the effects of surgical reconstruction. *Journal of the Medical Association of Thailand,* **83** (7), 708-718.

4 Davidson, J.H., Khor, K.E. & Jones, L.E. (2010) A cross-sectional study of post-amputation pain in upper and lower limb amputees, experience of a tertiary referral amputee clinic. *Disability & Rehabilitation,* **32** (22), 1855-1862.

5 Pool, J.L., Clark, W.D., Hudson, P. & Lombardo, M. (1956) Steroid hormonal response to stimulation of electrodes implanted in the subfrontal parts of the brain. In: Fields *et al.* (eds.), *Hypothalamic Hypophyseal Interrelationships,* pp. 114-124. Charles C. Thomas, Springfield, IL.

6 Mark, V.H. & Ervin, F.R. (1965) Role of thalamotomy in treatment of chronic severe pain. *Postgraduate Medicine,* **37**, 563-571.

7 Hosobuchi, Y., Adams, J.E. & Rutkin, B. (1973) Chronic thalamic stimulation for the control of facial anesthesia dolorosa. *Archives of Neurology,* **29** (3), 158-161.

8 Bittar, R.G., Kar-Purkayastha, I., Owen, S.L. *et al.* (2005) Deep brain stimulation for pain relief: a meta-analysis. *Journal of Clinical Neuroscience,* **12** (5), 515-519.

9 May, A., Bahra, A., Buchel, C. *et al.* (1998) Hypothalamic activation in cluster headache attacks. *Lancet,* **352** (9124), 275-278.

10 Richardson, D.E. & Akil, H. (1977) Long term results of periventricular gray self-stimulation. *Neurosurgery,* **1** (2), 199-202.

11 Plotkin, R. (1980) Deep-brain stimulation for the treatment of intractable pain. *South African Journal of Surgery,* **18** (4), 153-155.

12 Shulman, R., Turnbull, I.M., & Diewold, P. (1982) Psychiatric aspects of thalamic stimulation for neuropathic pain. *Pain,* **13** (2), 127-135.

13 Young, R.F., Kroening, R., Fulton, W. *et al.* (1985) Electrical stimulation of the brain in treatment of chronic pain. Experience over 5 years. *Journal of Neurosurgery,* **62** (3):389-96.

14 Hosobuchi, Y. (1986) Subcortical electrical stimulation for control of intractable pain in humans. Report of 122 cases (1970-1984). *Journal of Neurosurgery,* **64** (4), 543-553.

15 Levy, R.M., Lamb, S. & Adams, J.E. (1987) Treatment of chronic pain by deep brain stimulation: long term follow-up and review of the literature. *Neurosurgery,* **21** (6), 885-893.

16 Siegfried, J. (1987) Sensory thalamic neurostimulation for chronic pain. *Pacing Clinical Electrophysiology,* **10** (1 Pt 2), 209-212.

17 Gybels, J., Kupers, R. & Nuttin, B. (1993) Therapeutic stereotactic procedures on the thalamus for pain. *Acta Neurochirurgica (Wien),* **124** (1), 19-22.

18 Kumar, K., Toth, C. & Nath, R.K. (1997) Deep brain stimulation for intractable pain: a 15-year experience. *Neurosurgery,* **40** (4), 736-746; discussion 746-747.

19 Owen, S.L., Green, A.L., Stein, J.F. & Aziz, T.Z. (2006) Deep brain stimulation for the alleviation of post-stroke neuropathic pain. *Pain,* **120** (1-2), 202-206.

20 Hamani, C., Schwalb, J.M., Rezai, A.R. *et al.* (2006) Deep brain stimulation for chronic neuropathic pain: long-term outcome and the incidence of insertional effect. *Pain,* **125** (1-2): 188-196.

Chapter 12

Deep Brain Stimulation in Cluster Headache

Giovanni Broggi[1,2], Giuseppe Messina[1], and Angelo Franzini[1]

[1]Fondazione Instituto Neurologico "Carlo Besta", Milan, Italy
[2]Ludes University, Lugano, Switzerland

Introduction

Cluster headache is characterized by disabling, strictly unilateral painful attacks mostly perceived in the retro-orbital area. These headaches are accompanied by autonomic signs such as miosis, lacrimation, conjunctival injection, nasal congestion, and rhinorrhea. The prevalence of this disorder is estimated to be <1%, and it mostly affects males (male–female ratio between 2.5 and 7.1). The lifetime prevalence is 124 cases per 100 000 people and a 1-year prevalence is 53 cases per 100 000 people. Pain attacks typically last 15–180 min, occur daily, and are continuous or spaced out by remission periods of <1 month. In contrast, in the episodic form, attacks occur during a period ("cluster period") of 6–12 weeks interrupted by remission periods lasting up to 12 months.

Conventional conservative treatment of the chronic form of (chronic cluster headache, CCH) consists of prophylactic therapy (verapamil, methysergide, lithium carbonate, melatonin, gabapentin, sodium valproate, and corticosteroids) and abortive therapy (triptans, inhaled 100% oxygen, indomethacin, and opiates). In 10–20% of patients with CCH, conservative therapy does not satisfactorily control the symptoms, and so pain attacks become severely debilitating.

Neurostimulation: Principles and Practice, First Edition. Edited by Sam Eljamel and Konstantin V. Slavin.
© 2013 John Wiley & Sons, Ltd. Published 2013 by John Wiley & Sons, Ltd.

Rationale of deep brain stimulation in chronic cluster headache

DBS of the posterior hypothalamus (pHyp) was the first application in which the choice of target was motivated by functional neuroimaging data. Activation of the pHyp during cluster headache pain attacks was observed during PET in a previous study by May and co-workers [1]; this observation led to placement of DBS electrodes within the pHyp to inhibit the pathologically activated neuronal pools in patients with this disease.

To date, only a few papers have dealt with the electrophysiological properties of pHyp neurons in pain and behavior disorders. Moreover, just a few have attempted to quantify the firing discharge properties of this target. Microrecordings within the pHyp were performed in proximity to the stereotactic coordinates as suggested by us in 2003–specifically, 2 mm lateral to the midline, 3 mm posterior to the midcommissural point, and 5 mm below the commissural plane. Differences occurred in the mean firing rate (range 13-35 Hz). The firing discharge did not show variations for tactile, motor, autonomic, and emotional stimulations in all of the tested neurons.

Referral criteria

Initial guidelines for inclusion criteria for DBS of the pHyp in CCH were proposed by Leone *et al.* [2]: (1) the presence of diagnostic criteria for CCH according to the International Headache Society; (2) inadequate relief from prophylactic therapy, including verapamil, lithium, sodium valproate, methysergide, topiramate, gabapentin, non-steroidal anti-inflammatory drugs such as indomethacin, and corticosteroids; and (3) CCH lasting at least 2 years, with strictly lateralized pain attacks. Sillay and coworkers [3] expanded these criteria by including: (1) at least six debilitating headache episodes per week rated by patients as at least six on a visual analogue scale of 1-10; (2) unsatisfactory relief from abortive therapy, including oxygen, sumatriptan, and opioids; (3) failure of occipital nerve stimulation therapy for at least 1 year; and (4) completion of daily headache diaries over a period of 1 month prior to surgery. The last criterion should be considered as strictly dependent on the design of the study that these authors performed in 2009.

Most common programming parameters

The parameters used for chronic electrical stimulation were as follows: frequency 185 Hz, pulse width 60-90 μs, amplitude 1-3 V in unipolar configuration (case as anode). The IPG was turned on a few days after the intervention in all of the patients, and the stimulation amplitude was progressively increased but remained below the threshold for adverse effects.

Evidence to date

DBS in CCH remains experimental. In our entire series, 71% of the postoperative days were pain free, and the intensity and duration of pain bouts were
significantly reduced. The overall drug dosage was reduced to <20% of the
preoperative levels. The mean time to pain freedom or reduction was 42
days (1–86 days); the mean amplitude of stimulation used was 2.4 V (0.6–
3.3 V). The mean follow-up was 4 years; after the first 2 years of clinical
follow-up, major improvement in pain or pain disappearance was observed
in 15 (94%) of 16 patients. After a mean of 4 years of follow-up, a state of
persistent freedom from painful attacks was still present in 10 patients
(62%). Four patients (25%) still required prophylactic drugs to prevent pain
attacks. In the last 2 years of follow-up three patients no longer benefited
from stimulation despite several changes in the parameters. In these three
patients, the disease turned from the chronic form to the episodic form
(that is, periods of complete remission lasting several months alternating
with periods of attacks). With the series reported earlier taken as a whole,
the percentage of patients considered to be responders to DBS surgery is
63% [4,5,6].

Conclusions

Data suggest that the pHyp interacts with different neural networks that
have a link or a common path in this small volume of brain. In particular,
to understand the possibly involved neurophysiological circuits we must
note the following phenomena involved in pHyp DBS: the neurovegetative
responses linked to the pain threshold of the ipsilateral orbital region (CCH,
SUNCT (short-lasting unilateral neuralgiform headache attacks with conjunctival injection and tearing), and blood pressure regulation); the effect on
cortical excitability and reticular system (multifocal epilepsy, psychomotor
agitation, and sleep); the behavioral responses (rage, aggressiveness, and
disruptive behavior).

From these data we can argue that the pHyp modulates different neurological functions, and its dysregulation can result in a consistent variety of
neurological symptoms. Unfortunately, data are still not sufficient to build
up a specific theory that could define the precise role of the pHyp, although
we can hypothesize that it controls relationships between the neurophysiological circuits involved in pain behavior and the neurovegetative system.
Furthermore, during pHyp DBS no endocrine changes have been demonstrated, and so we must consider that the functions of this area are independent from the classic hormonal mechanisms controlled by the more
anterior hypothalamic nuclei. Another relevant point is related to the latency
periods that elapse between the beginning of stimulation and the appearance
of therapeutic effects.

This phenomenon has been highlighted by a French multicenter study, where turning the stimulator on and off at 1-month intervals resulted in an ineffectiveness in the control of pain in patients with CCH; after 1 year of continuous stimulation in the same group of patients the therapeutic effect developed as in other reported series in the literature.

We hypothesize that pHyp DBS acts through the remodeling of neural circuits and so it requires a certain amount of time conditioned by individual neural plasticity. Similar mechanisms may be called upon to explain the time-related effects of pallidal DBS in dystonia or the latency between the start of stimulation and the therapeutic effects in depressed patients treated with subgenu chronic stimulation.

References

1 May, A., Bahra, A., Büchel, C. *et al.* (1998) Hypothalamic activation in cluster headache attacks. *Lancet*, **352** (9124), 275-278.

2 Leone, M., Franzini, A. & Bussone, G. (2001) Stereotactic stimulation of posterior hypothalamic gray matter in a patient with intractable cluster headache. *The New England Journal of Medicine*, **345** (19), 1428-1429

3 Sillay, K.A., Sani, S. & Starr, P.A. (2010) Deep brain stimulation for medically intractable cluster headache. *Neurobiology of Disease*, **38** (3), 361-368.

4 Fontaine, D., Lazorthes, Y., Mertens, P. *et al.* (2010) Safety and efficacy of deep brain stimulation in refractory cluster headache: a randomized placebo-controlled double-blind trial followed by a 1-year open extension. *The Journal of Headache and Pain*, **11** (1), 23-31.

5 Franzini, A., Messina, G., Cordella, R. *et al.* (2010) Deep brain stimulation of the posteromedial hypothalamus: indications, long-term results, and neurophysiological considerations. *Neurosurgical Focus*, **29** (2), E13.

6 Schoenen, J., Di Clemente, L., Vandenheede, M. *et al.* (2005) Hypothalamic stimulation in chronic cluster headache: a pilot study of efficacy and mode of action. *Brain: A Journal of Neurology*, **128** (Pt 4), 940-947.

Part 2
Vagus Nerve Stimulation

Chapter 13

Mechanism of Action and Overview of Vagus Nerve Stimulation Technology

Sam Eljamel

University of Dundee, Ninewells Hospital and Medical School, Dundee, UK

Mechanism of action

The exact mechanism of vagus nerve stimulation (VNS) is not fully understood. The proposed mechanism of action of VNS includes:

(1) Alteration of epinephrine release by projections of solitary tract to locus coeruleus in the medulla oblongata.
(2) Elevation of gamma aminobutyric acid (GABA) levels in the brain stem.
(3) Inhibition of aberrant cortical activity by reticular formation in the brain stem [1].
(4) Desynchronizing electroencephalographic activity was also thought to play a role in how VNS works [2,3].
(5) Blood flow studies had also revealed increased cerebral blood flow in the dorsal medulla oblongata, hypothalamus, and the insula and decrease of blood flow in the hippocampus, the amygdala, and the cingulate gyrus [3,4,5,6].

It was initially thought that stimulation at higher thresholds, C-fibers in the vagus nerve were responsible for the antiseizure effect although this is now considered to be incorrect, with larger, low-threshold A and B fibers thought to be involved instead [7,8,9]. Animal studies using c-fos gene activation have suggested involvement of the amygdala, which is highly epileptogenic; the habenula and posteromedian nucleus of the thalamus, which are involved in seizure regulation; and the locus coeruleus and A5 nuclei of the brainstem,

Neurostimulation: Principles and Practice, First Edition. Edited by Sam Eljamel and Konstantin V. Slavin.
© 2013 John Wiley & Sons, Ltd. Published 2013 by John Wiley & Sons, Ltd.

which all appear to be activated during VNS [10]. Likewise, lesioning the locus coeruleus also appears to inhibit the effects of VNS by limiting norepine-phrine (noradrenaline) release [11], while altering GABA release or glutamate transmission in the NTS can also influence seizure activity [12]. These studies are technically challenging, particularly the difficulty in controlling the secondary effects of VNS in c-*fos* experiments, but they do suggest strongly that the NTS and its cortical projections are critical in the anticonvulsant effects of VNS. A summary of these, and other hypotheses, was prepared by Binnie [13] in his review of VNS in 2000. Equally VNS imparts its antidepression effects through these connections to the limbic system. It is difficult to imagine a single mechanism responsible for VNS effects and it is more likely many mechanisms are at play; by altering the electric charge in the NTS, the brain circuits connected to the NTS are therefore modulated in one way or another to prevent seizure activity, prevent spread of seizures, alter the nature of the seizure and alter the harmonic frequency of these oscillators.

Overview of vagus nerve stimulation indications

Approved VNS indications include treatment refractory epilepsy and treatment refractory major depression.

Vagus nerve stimulation in treatment refractory epilepsy

Epilepsy prevalence is 2–5% worldwide (World Health Organization estimate). About 5–30% of people with epilepsy have medically refractory complex partial seizures [14]. VNS was approved by the FDA (US Food and Drug Administration) in 1997 as an adjunctive therapy for epilepsy in adults over 12 years of age with partial onset seizures.

The National Institute for Health and Clinical Excellence in the UK issued its guidance in 2004 regarding VNS in refractory epilepsy in children. VNS is a viable option to reduce the severity and shorten the duration of seizures in those patients who remain refractory despite optimal drug therapy or surgical intervention, as well as in those with debilitating side effects of antiepileptic medications; this was demonstrated in randomized controlled trials [15,16,17,18] and uncontrolled retrospective studies [19,20].

Post-marketing experience suggested improved seizure control over time [19,20,21]. In children younger than 12 years of age, 46% experienced more than 50% reduction in seizure frequency at their most recent visit, and in another study of 28 children younger than 12 years of age, a mean reduction of 62% was reported in seizure frequency at 1 year [22,23,24,25]. There was also evidence to suggest that quality of life improved as a result of the procedure. Forty-eight percent of patients or carers thought that alertness was better or much better after 3 months [22,23,24,25]. Table 13.1 summarizes the advantages and disadvantages of VNS in epilepsy. For details see Chapter 14.

Table 13.1 Advantages and disadvantages of vagal nerve stimulation in epilepsy

Advantages	Disadvantages
Extracranial procedure with no risks associated with respective epilepsy surgery	Only a small number of patients become seizure free
Reduction of 50% of seizures in 50% of patients with treatment refractory partial complex seizures	Efficacy is difficult to predict before VNS implantation
Patient may have some control over seizures by hand-held magnet	Battery changes are inevitable and batteries deplete without warning
Treatment compliance is ensured	Risk of hoarseness and dysphonia
No interactions with anticonvulsant medications	Risk of coughing and tickly throat
Well tolerated and accepted treatment by patients	Relatively high cost for devices

Vagal nerve stimulation in treatment refractory major depression

Major depression is a major public health problem worldwide with a lifetime prevalence of 13% and 12-month prevalence of 5%. Among those who have suffered one major depressive episode, approximately three-quarters will have a recurrent episode and many will not achieve remission [26,27]. One-third of those suffering major depression fail first antidepressive therapy and 20% become resistant to lithium, combination therapy, psychotherapy, and electroconvulsive therapy [28]. The FDA approved VNS for treatment-resistant depression in 2005. A review of 18 studies including one randomized controlled trial with 1251 VNS-treated patients with treatment-resistant depression reported reduction of 50% or more in the Hamilton Depression Rating Scale (HAMD) from baseline scores ranging from 31% to 40% of patients in up to 10-week follow-up and in 27% to 58% of patients in 12-month or more follow-up. A case series of 74 patients with severe depression (>2 years or at least four depressive episodes) reported that mean HAMD scores improved significantly compared with baseline at 12-month follow-up ($p < 0.0001$), and that 55% of patients had a response to VNS and 50 of 264 patients with treatment-resistant depression responded [29,30,31,32,33,34,35]. Table 13.2 summarizes the efficacy of VNS in treatment refractory depression. For a more detailed account of the evidence please refer to Chapter 15.

Side effects of vagal nerve therapy

Adverse events (AEs) related to VNS treatment of epilepsy were hoarseness (56%), paresthesia (29%), dyspnea (27%), coughing (23%), throat pain (8%), headache (8%), hypophonia (4%), vocal cord paralysis (4%), sensation of throat constriction (2%), abdominal pain (2%), jaw pain (2%), double

Table 13.2 Summary of vagal nerve stimulation efficacy in treatment refractory depression

Time from VNS	3 months	6 months	9 months	1 year
Response rate (%)*	30–36	39–44	46–53	47–55
Remission (%)*	11–18	15–25	26–28	28–33

*Response rate is defined as reduction of 50% or more on the Hamilton Depression Rating Scale (HAMD-28) and remission means HAMD-28 score of 10 or less.

Table 13.3 Risks and side effects of vagal nerve stimulation

Risk/side effect	VNS in epilepsy (%)	VNS in depression (%)
Hoarseness	56	63
Paresthesia	29	18
Dyspnea	27	10
Coughing	23	26
Throat pain	8	20
Headache	8	3.3
Jaw pain	2	2
Infection	2	2
Dysphonia	4	4
Suicide	N/A	3.3
Attempted suicide	N/A	1.6

vision (2%), flushing (2%), and agitation (2%). Eight patients (17%) did not present any AEs related to VNS treatment. Most AEs were reported in the first year of VNS treatment and resolved over time. In some cases, AEs briefly recurred after generator replacement, especially when VNS was interrupted for 3 weeks. Stimulation-induced pain or discomfort in the neck/throat area occurred initially during ramp-up in most new patients. Symptoms resolved immediately as current output, pulse width, or frequency was reduced to previously tolerated settings [36].

AEs related to VNS treatment of resistant depression occurred in 17% of patients, including two patients with worsening depression and one with myocardial infarction. In six short-term studies two patients discontinued VNS treatment because of adverse events. In the case series of 74 patients, 2% of 61 patients available at 6-month follow-up were reported to have committed suicide. In a randomized controlled trial one of 112 VNS-treated patients was reported to have committed suicide. In the case series of 74 patients 1% of patients developed a manic episode, 1% had worsening depression, 10% had dyspnea, and 20% reported pain at 3-month follow-up. In the same study, the most common adverse events were cough and voice alteration (26% and 63% of patients, respectively, at 3 months; $n = 70$). Hypomania or mania was reported after VNS treatment in five patients across two case series (including 317 VNS-treated patients) [29,30,31,32,33,34,35]. Table 13.3 summarizes the risks and side effects of VNS in epilepsy and depression.

Vagal nerve stimulation components

VNS consists of components surgically implanted by the surgeon and external components to communicate with the implanted device.

The implantable components consist of

(1) A pulse generator (NCP) houses the battery and electronic components that regulate the stimulation parameters (Figure 13.1). The most recent model (Demipulse™ Model 103) compatible with single pin leads, weighs 16 g, and 6.9 × 45 × 32 mm in size. Its dual pin model 104 is designed for replacing older and larger NCPs with dual pin leads (Table 13.4).

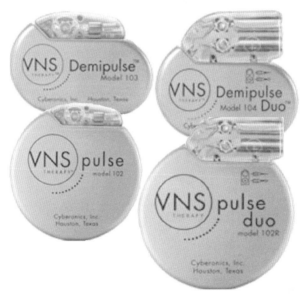

Figure 13.1 Photograph of four models of NCPs: Demipulse™ Model 103 (top left) with single pin, Demipulse™ Model 104 Duo (top right) with dual pins, pulse model 102 and pulse duo model 102R (bottom left and right) older models.

Table 13.4 Comparison of NCP models

NCP model	102	102R	103	104
Size (mm)	6.9 × 52.2 × 51.6	6.9 × 58.9 × 51.6	6.9 × 45 × 32	6.9 × 45 × 39
Weight (g)	25	27	16	17
Heather	Single pin	Dual pins	Single pin	Dual pins
Compatible leads	302 and 303	300	302 and 303	300
Battery type	Lithium carbon	Lithium Carbon	Lithium carbon	Lithium carbon
Expected longevity (years)	6	6	6	6

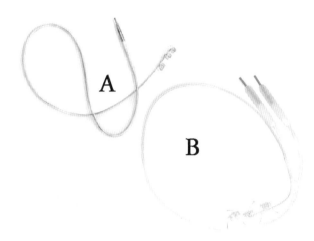

Figure 13.2 Photograph of the vagal nerve stimulation leads: (A) single pin for NCP models 102 and 103; (B) dual pins for NCP models 102R and 104.

Table 13.5 Vagal nerve stimulation leads

Lead model	Inner helical diameter (mm)	Length (cm)	Resistance (ohms)	Compatible NCP
302-20	2	43	180–250	102 and 103
302-30	3	43	180–250	102 and 103
303-20	2	43	180–250	102 and 103
303-30	3	43	180–250	102 and 103
304-20	2	43	120–180	102 and 103
304-30	3	43	120–180	102 and 103

(2) A wire wrapped around the left vagus nerve (lead). The lead consists of helical contacts that wrap around the left vagus nerve with an anchor (Figure 13.2). Dual-pin leads (B) are no longer distributed. Available leads are summarized in Table 13.5.

The NCP is implanted in the left upper chest wall just below the collar bone (clavicle) or in the left axilla. The NCP provides vagus stimulation via the lead (Figure 13.3).

The non-implantable VNS components consist of:

(1) Programming wand

The programming wand is a hand-held device that transmits programming and interrogation information between a VNS Therapy Computer and the VNS Therapy Pulse Generator (NCP). The wand is held over the NCP during interrogation and programming of the NCP (Figure 13.4).

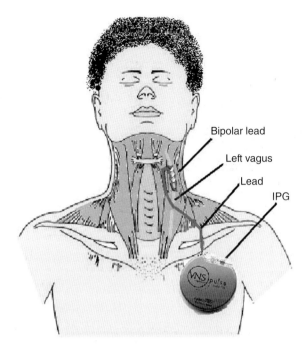

Figure 13.3 Diagram showing location of the vagal nerve stimulation implant. IPG, implantable pulse generator.

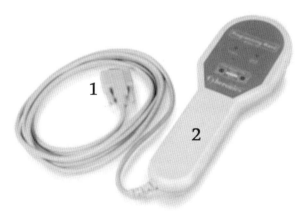

Figure 13.4 Vagal nerve stimulation (VNS) programming wand model 201; 2, the wand placed over the NCP; 1, serial connection to connect to VNS programming computer or hand-held device.

(2) Physician programmer

This is a laptop computer or a hand-held device that connects to the programming wand and runs VNS programming software. The software allows physicians to interrogate and read the VNS therapy parameters and transmit new parameters into the device. The physician using the VNS programmer is able to change pulse width, amplitude, frequency, and duration of VNS stimulation (Figure 13.5).

(3) Patient's magnet

The magnet is worn by patients with VNS to enable them to reset the NCP, test the daily function of the VNS, temporarily inhibit VNS therapy, or provide on-demand VNS therapy (Figure 13.6).

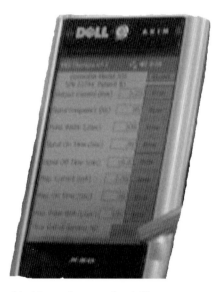

Figure 13.5 Hand-held vagal nerve simulation programmer.

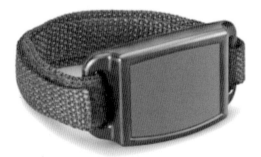

Figure 13.6 Patient's magnet model 220.

References

1 Ghanem, T. & Early, S.V. (2006) Vagal nerve stimulator implantation: an otolaryngologist's perspective. *Otolaryngology–Head and Neck Surgery: Official Journal of American Academy of Otolaryngology-Head and Neck Surgery*, **135** (1), 46–51.

2 Henry, T. (2002) Therapeutic mechanisms of vagus nerve stimulation. *Neurology*, **59** (6 Suppl.), S3–S14.

3 Koo, B. (2001) EEG changes with vagus nerve stimulation. *Journal of Clinical Neurophysiology*, **18**, 434–441.

4 Ng, M. & Devinsky, O. (2004) Vagus nerve stimulation for refractory idiopathic generalized epilepsy. *Seizure: The Journal of the British Epilepsy Association*, **13**, 176–178.

5 Schachter, S. (2002) Vagus nerve stimulation therapy summary: five years after FDA approval. *Neurology*, **59**, S15–S20.

6 Sucholeiki, R., Alsaadi, T.M., Morris, G.L., III, *et al.* (2002) fMRI in patients implanted with a vagal nerve stimulator. *Seizure: The Journal of the British Epilepsy Association*, **11**, 157–162.

7 Krahl, S.E., Senanayake, S.S. & Handforth, A. (2001) Destruction of peripheral C-fibers does not alter subsequent vagus nerve stimulation-induced seizure suppression in rats. *Epilepsia*, **42** (5), 586–589.

8 Koo, B., Ham, S.D., Sood, S. & Tarver, B. (2001) Human vagus nerve electrophysiology: a guide to vagus nerve stimulation parameters. *Journal of Clinical Neurophysiology: Official Publication of the American Electroencephalographic Society*, **18** (5), 429–433.

9 Chase, M.H., Sterman, M.B. & Clemente, C.D. (1966) Cortical and subcortical patterns of response to afferent vagal stimulation. *Experimental Neurology*, **16** (1), 36–49.

10 Naritoku, D.K., Terry, W.J. & Helfert, R.H. (1995) Regional induction of fos immunoreactivity in the brain by anticonvulsant stimulation of the vagus nerve. *Epilepsy Research*, **22** (1), 53–62.

11 Krahl, S.E., Clark, K.B., Smith, D.C. & Browning, R.A. (1998) Locus coeruleus lesions suppress the seizure-attenuating effects of vagus nerve stimulation. *Epilepsia*, **39** (7), 709–714.

12 Walker, B.R., Easton, A. & Gale, K. (1999) Regulation of limbic motor seizures by GABA and glutamate transmission in nucleus tractus solitarius. *Epilepsia*, **40** (8), 1051–1057.

13 Binnie, C.D. (2000) Vagus nerve stimulation for epilepsy: a review. *Seizure: The Journal of the British Epilepsy Association*, **9** (3), 161–169.

14 Bryant, J. & Stein, K. (1998) Vagus nerve stimulation in epilepsy. DEC Report No. 82. Wessex Institute for Health Research and Development, University of Southampton, Southampton, UK.

15 Ben-Menachem, E., Mañon-Espaillat, R., Ristanovic, R. *et al.* (1994) Vagus nerve stimulation for treatment of partial seizures: 1. A controlled study of effects on seizures. *Epilepsia*, **35**, 616–626.

16 Ramsay, R.E., Uthman, B.M., Augustinsson, L.E. *et al.* (1994) Vagus nerve stimulation for treatment of partial seizures: 2. Safety, side effects, and tolerability. *Epilepsia*, **35**, 627–636.

17 Handforth, A., DeGiorgio, C.M., Schachter, S.C. *et al.* (1998) Vagus nerve stimulation therapy for partial-onset seizures. A randomized active-control trial. *Neurology*, **51**, 48–54.

18 DeGiorgio, C., Schachter, S., Handforth, A. *et al.* (2000) Prospective long-term study of Vagus Nerve Stimulation for the treatment of refractory seizures. *Epilepsia*, **41**, 1195-1200.

19 Ben-Menachem, E., Hellstroem, K., Waldton, C. & Augustinsson, L.E. (1999) Evaluation of refractory epilepsy treated with vagus nerve stimulation for up to 5 years. *Neurology*, **52**, 1265-1267.

20 Hui, A.C., Lam, J.M., Wong, K.S. *et al.* (2004) Vagus nerve stimulation for refractory epilepsy: long term efficacy and side-effects. *Chinese Medical Journal*, **117**, 58-61.

21 Morris, G.L., III, Mueller, W.M. & Vagus Nerve Stimulation Study Group E01-E05 (1999) Long-term treatment with vagus nerve stimulation in patients with refractory epilepsy. *Neurology*, **53**, 1731-1735.

22 Buoni, S., Mariottini, A., Pieri, S. *et al.* (2004) VNS for drug resistant epilepsy in children and young adults. *Brain and Development*, **26** (3), 158-163.

23 DeGiorgio, C., Heck, C., Bunch, S. *et al.* (2005) Vagus nerve stimulation for epilepsy: randomized comparison of three stimulation paradigms. *Neurology*, **65**, 317-319.

24 Smyth, M., Tubbs, R., Bebin, E. *et al.* (2003) Complications of chronic VNS for epilepsy in children. *Journal of Neurosurgery*, **99** (3), 500-503.

25 Zamponi, N., Rychlicki, F., Cardinali, C. *et al.* (2002) Intermittent vagal nerve stimulation in pediatric patients: 1-year follow up. *Child's Nervous System*, **18** (1-2), 61-66.

26 Hasin, D.S., Goodwin, R.D., Stinson, F.S. & Grant, B.F. (2005) Epidemiology of major depressive disorder: results from the National Epidemiologic Survey on Alcoholism and Related Conditions. *Archives of General Psychiatry*, **62** (10), 1097-1106.

27 Mann, J.J. (2005) The medical management of depression. *The New England Journal of Medicine*, **353** (17), 1819-1834.

28 Keller, M.B. (2005) Issues in treatment-resistant depression. *The Journal of Clinical Psychiatry*, **66** (Suppl. 8), 5-12.

29 Rush, A.J., George, M.S., Sackheim, H.A. *et al.* (2000) Vagus nerve stimulation (VNS) for treatment-resistant depressions: a multicenter study. *Biological Psychiatry*, **47** (4), 276-286.

30 Marangell, L.B., Rush, A.J., George, M.S. *et al.* (2002) Vagus nerve stimulation (VNS) for major depressive episodes: one year outcomes. *Biological Psychiatry*, **51** (4), 280-287.

31 Sackheim, H.A., Rush, A.J., George, M.S. *et al.* (2001) Vagus nerve stimulation (VNS) for treatment-resistant depression: efficacy, side effects, and predictors of outcome. *Neuropsychopharmacology*, **25** (5), 713-728.

32 Nahas, Z., Marangell, L.B., Husain, M.M. *et al.* (2005) Two-year outcome of vagus nerve stimulation (VNS) for treatment of major depressive episodes. *The Journal of Clinical Psychiatry*, **66** (9), 1097-1104.

33 Rush, A.J., Marangell, L.B., Sackheim, H.A. *et al.* (2005) Vagus nerve stimulation for treatment-resistant depression: a randomized, controlled acute phase trial. *Biological Psychiatry*, **58** (5), 347-354.

34 Rush, A.J., Sackheim, H.A., Marangell, L.B. *et al.* (2005) Effects of 12 months of vagus nerve stimulation in treatment-resistant depression: a naturalistic study. *Biological Psychiatry*, **58** (5), 355-363.

35 George, M.S., Rush, A.J., Marangell, L.B. *et al.* (2005) A one-year comparison of vagus nerve stimulation with treatment as usual for treatment-resistant depression. *Biological Psychiatry*, **58** (5), 364-373.

36 Uthman, B.M., Reichl, A.M., Dean, J.C. *et al.* (2004) Effectiveness of VNS stimulation in epilepsy patients, A 12 years observation. *Neurology*, **63**, 1124-1126.

Chapter 14
Vagus Nerve Stimulation in Epilepsy

Ian Morrison

Ninewells Hospital and Medical School, Dundee, UK

Introduction

Epilepsy is a common condition, affecting between five and eight per 1000 of the general population in developed countries [1]. Despite an ever-increasing number of drugs available for its treatment, studies suggest that over a third of patients will be refractory to drug treatment and continue to have unacceptable seizures or intolerable side effects from their anticonvulsants [2,3].

Non-pharmacological treatments are available for these medically refractory patients, including ketogenic diets, cerebellar stimulation, thalamic stimulation, and resective surgery. While DBS for epilepsy was covered in Chapter 8, it is widely accepted that the most effective treatment is resective surgery. However, not all patients are suitable for this intervention and in this setting, vagus nerve stimulation (VNS) can be considered as an alternative [4].

The rationale for vagus nerve stimulation in epilepsy

Historical background

Some of the earliest experiments in VNS to control seizures were undertaken in the 1880s by an American neurologist, James Leonard Corning. At the time, facial flushing and increased carotid artery pulsation were thought to represent "venous hyperaemia" of the central nervous system and that

Neurostimulation: Principles and Practice, First Edition. Edited by Sam Eljamel and Konstantin V. Slavin.
© 2013 John Wiley & Sons, Ltd. Published 2013 by John Wiley & Sons, Ltd.

compression of the carotid artery, or even its ligation, may be a method of controlling epilepsy. To refine this technique, Corning undertook a number of uncontrolled experiments looking at direct carotid compression and also transcutaneous electrical stimulation of the vagus nerve to control cerebral blood flow and reduce the number of seizures. This early form of VNS was successful but was not widely adopted by his colleagues and soon fell out of favor [5].

A variety of experiments since the 1930s have shown, mainly in cat models, that VNS can result in changes in electroencephalograms (EEGs), and in particular desynchronize EEGs, or block interictal spiking. EEG desynchronization that occurs with arousal has been shown to block interictal epileptiform activity on EEG, while hypersynchrony is often associated with epileptic discharges. It was therefore reasonable to test VNS as a potential therapy for epilepsy and Zabara [6], in 1985 using a strychnine-induced seizure model in the dog, was the first to demonstrate that VNS could rapidly suppress seizures. Reduction in seizure frequency or severity with VNS was later confirmed in seizure models in both rats and monkeys, leading to the first human pilot studies in 1990 [7,8].

Vagus nerve anatomy

The vagus nerve is the longest cranial nerve and studies in the cat have shown that it is a mixed nerve, with 20% of fibers providing parasympathetic innervation from the nucleus ambiguus and the dorsal motor nucleus of the vagus nerve to the heart, gastrointestinal (GI) tract and lungs, in addition to the voluntary muscles of the larynx and pharynx. Although both vagus nerves develop symmetrically initially, rotation of the abdominal and thoracic organs during embryonic development results in the right vagus nerve becoming associated with the cardiac atria (and sinoatrial node), liver, and duodenum, and the left with the cardiac ventricles (and atrioventricular node) and fundus of the stomach. As a consequence, the left vagus nerve is stimulated in VNS to avoid unwanted bradycardia. However, it also contains 80% afferent fibers, providing visceral sensation from receptors in the head, thorax, abdomen, and colon. Receptors are found in a number of locations, including the lungs, concha of the ear, GI tract, heart, and aorta, with their afferent fibers projecting, via their cell bodies in the jugular and nodose ganglia to the nucleus tractus solitarius (NTS) [9,10]. The NTS has a number of output pathways to autonomic preganglionic and related somatic motor neurons in the medulla and the spinal cord to control cardiovascular homeostasis; the reticular formation of the medulla to control various autonomic and respiratory reflexes; and an ascending projection to the forebrain, the majority of which travels via the parabrachial nucleus. The parabrachial nucleus has connections to several parts of the brain that could be involved in modulating cortical activity, which could also have an influence on seizure activity. For example, projections extend to the insular cortex, via the ventroposterior parvocellular nucleus; the intralaminar nuclei of the thalamus, which has connections throughout the cerebral cortex; and projections for visceral supply to the hypothalamus, amygdala and basal forebrain [11].

Mechanism of action

The mechanism of action of VNS is clearly different from that of anticonvulsant drugs, whose effects are mediated via neurotransmitters, receptor binding sites, or neuronal membrane conductance. The pathways involved in seizure control with VNS, however, remain unclear. The current hypotheses are covered in Chapter 13 and Table 14.1.

Patient selection and referral criteria

There is good evidence that patients with refractory epilepsy respond well to resective surgery, which can be curative, if selected appropriately.

Table 14.1 Experimental evidence suggesting potential sites of vagal nerve stimulation (VNS) action (adapted from Binnie [12])

Potential modes of action VNS
Functional anatomy
Multiple projection pathways identified, through nucleus of the tractus solitarius to:
locus coeruleus, parabrachial nucleus, dorsal raphe, nucleus ambiguus, cerebellum, hypothalamus, thalamus insula, medullary reticular formation, substantia innominata, zona incerta
Lesioning/inactivation of locus coeruleus reduces the anticonvulsant effect
Positron emission tomography
Blood flow increased in rostral medulla, right post-central gyrus, hypothalami, thalami, insulae, cerebellum
Blood flow decreased in hippocampi, amygdalae, posterior cinguli [2]
Electrophysiology
EEG desynchronized or synchronized in cat   Little effect in man
Evoked potential latencies increased in man   A- and B-fiber dependent [6], or no effect
Neurochemistry
Serotoninergic: CSF 5-hydroxyindole acetic acid increase
Serotoninergic: Activation of locus coeruleus
Dopaminergic: CSF homovanillic acid elevated
GABAergic: GABA or glutamate dependent. CSF GABA elevated
VNS induces *fos* production in superior colliculus, amygdala, cortex, post-lateral thalamus and hypothalamus

Evaluation of patients involves video-electroencephalogram (EEG) monitoring, high-field magnetic resonance imaging (MRI), single photon emission computed tomography scanning (where appropriate), and depth electrode EEG if necessary. This is also supported by extensive neuropsychological evaluation.

Unlike resective surgery, however, VNS is a palliative procedure rather than curative and should only be considered once a patient has been declared unsuitable for surgical resection. The only absolute contraindication to VNS is previous left or bilateral cervical vagotomy but relative contraindications include progressive stroke or other neurological illness, cardiac dysrhythmias, respiratory disease, and vasovagal syncope.

There have been reports that patients can experience swallowing difficulties following implantation, often leading to aspiration, and caution is advised in patients with pre-existing swallowing problems, particularly in children with severe motor disorders. Additionally, recent reports have suggested that VNS may cause abnormalities in sleep breathing, particularly in children with pre-existing respiratory problems. However, these reports have contradicted previous work that suggests VNS has no effect on sleep breathing, and, until this is clarified, further caution is advised in this patient group [13,14]. Likewise, there have been no studies looking at VNS in pregnancy, and, as a result, the manufacturers recommend that it should only be used "during pregnancy if clearly needed."

The initial Food and Drug Administration approval for VNS in the USA was for "adjunctive therapy in reducing the frequency of seizures in adults and adolescents over 12 years of age with partial onset seizures, which are refractory to antiepileptic medications." Similar guidelines exist from the National Institute for Health and Clinical Excellence in the UK, although it cautions that the procedure should only be undertaken in children by specialist pediatric epilepsy teams.

Evidence to date

Two studies have shown the effect of VNS in humans over a 3-month period. The first trial, known as E03 was an international, multicenter trial of patients over 12 years old who had more than six partial seizures per month, despite treatment with appropriate anticonvulsants [15]. This study randomized patients into two groups: one with high stimulation VNS stimulation (30 s every 5 min of 30 Hz, 500 μs up to 3.5 mA) and low stimulation (30 s every 90 min, 1 Hz, 130 μs, <3.5 mA). This study showed that the high-stimulation group had a 24.5% reduction in seizures compared with 6.1% in the low-stimulation group ($p = 0.01$). Further, 31% of the high-stimulation group had a 50% or greater seizure reduction compared with 13% in the low-stimulation group. A second trial, E05, showed broadly similar results using a similar patient cohort and stimulation regimen (28% seizure reduction in the high-stimulation group, 15% in the low-stimulation group but no significant differ-ence in 50% seizure reduction) [16].

Longer-term studies, looking at the effects up to 3 years (E05 and E01-E05) have shown that the effect of VNS appears cumulative with time. Indeed, patients had a median seizure reduction of 45% at 1 year and 34% had a seizure reduction of 50% at 1 year (using a current of 1.7 mA). At 2 and 3 years, 50% seizure reduction was seen in 43%. Although no formal studies have been performed in children, there is considerable case report data suggesting comparable reductions in seizures to adults [17,18].

Although these studies looked at partial onset seizures, there is evidence (mainly from case reports) of benefit in tuberous sclerosis, status epilepticus, Unverricht-Lundborg myoclonic epilepsy, and infantile spasms. Likewise, there has been benefit in Lennox-Gastaut syndrome, and in particular with patients who have predominantly atonic seizures [19].

Common programming parameters

Once the device is implanted on the first occasion, programming the device is usually deferred for 1–2 weeks to allow recovery from the operation. It is not possible to establish a patient on a high output current initially, and instead a "ramping up" procedure is undertaken where the output current is slowly increased over a period of several weeks. Programming the device is non-invasive, using a programming "wand" connected to a computer (Figure 14.1B).

Unfortunately, optimum VNS settings, despite many years of clinical use, remain unknown. Initial human studies used "default" settings with a signal frequency of 30 Hz, a 500-μs pulse width, an on time of 30 s and an off time of 5 min.

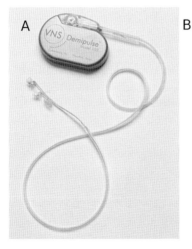
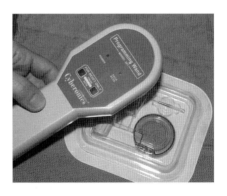

Figure 14.1 A, The vagus nerve stimulation system. B, The programming wand interrogating the device prior to implantation.

The extent of the depolarization of the nerve is dependent on the magnitude of the current delivered (output current) and duration of the stimulus (pulse width). If the pulse width remains unchanged, increasing the output current will depolarize large, low-threshold fibers initially, then smaller, high-threshold fibers later.

Early studies thought that C fibers were responsible for the antiseizure effects of VNS and, as a consequence, stimulation parameters used high output currents and pulse widths. However, this largely fell out of favor when it was realized that A and B fibers are likely to be most effective in controlling seizures, and stimulation of C fibers can cause unwanted autonomic side effects (including bradycardia). Current stimulation parameters are not thought to be sufficient to stimulate C fibers as a consequence.

The output current is started usually at 0.25 mA and increased every few weeks by 0.25-0.5 mA, depending on patient tolerance. The initial target range for the output current lies between 1.25 and 2 mA, although this is variable and largely dependent on patient tolerability and also clinical response with some patients requiring stimulation up to 3.5 mA. Children are known to have higher stimulation thresholds and lower conduction velocities in their vagus nerve than adults; therefore, a higher current (or longer pulse width) will be required in this population. There is no evidence to support further increases in output current in an effort to improve efficacy by stimulating higher threshold fibers, once a therapeutic response is achieved. Instead, this may actually be less well tolerated and provoke side effects in sensitive patients.

The pulse width can be altered with a range from 130 to 500 μs. If the pulse width duration is reduced, the ability to depolarize the nerve is reduced and a higher output current is required, with the potential to cause unwanted side effects. However, the relationship between output current and pulse width is non-linear, making it difficult to predict changes. For example, reducing the pulse width from 500 to 250 μs only requires a slight increase in output current but any further reduction, to 130 μs, for example, requires much higher output currents. These changes have been confirmed on functional MRI studies of activation. Clinically, most VNS devices are set to a pulse width of 500 μs. If the patient experiences side effects, the pulse width can be reduced to 250 μs. Although the efficacy remains largely unchanged, the reduced pulse width means this is often better tolerated. Reducing the pulse width to less than 250 μs is not widely undertaken and not recommended.

A number of other settings can be manipulated within the VNS. There is some evidence from animal studies that the optimum frequency for VNS is in the range of 10-60 Hz. However, studies in rat models have suggested that using low stimulus frequencies (less than 20 Hz) can preferentially stimulate slow conducting C fibers (that have a longer refractory period) and thus increase autonomic side effects. In humans, most clinicians therefore aim for settings between 20-30 Hz, although the evidence for this is limited and based largely on clinical experience.

Likewise, the on and off times of the stimulator can also be altered but again, there is no evidence to support which settings are best. The duty cycle of the device is measured as the: on time/on + off time in seconds). There is good evidence that duty cycles of less than 50% are safe, with some clinicians prefer a rapid cycling with an on time of 7 s and an off time of 18 s (duty cycle 28%), to maximize the amount of stimulation given on a daily basis. However, this has significant implications for battery life, which is substantially shortened using this regime. Another regime is similar to the default settings used in the initial studies, with an on time of 30 s and an off time of between 3 and 5 min (duty cycle 14 and 9% respectively), which provides less stimulation per day but can significantly prolong battery life. There is no evidence in difference in efficacy between the stimulation parameters, with lower duty cycles preferred initially. If a patient fails to respond, patients may be switched to higher duty cycles if tolerated.

Additionally, the patient or carers can be given a magnet, often worn on the wrist, to control the stimulation of the device. This can be used to initiate a burst of stimulation to terminate a single seizure or status. Again, there is no consensus on the optimum settings for this facility, but the usual current is delivered with the same pulse width, and the on time is prolonged to around 30 s.

Following the "ramping-up" period, patients are normally reviewed at 4- to 6-monthly intervals. During these review sessions, the device can be interrogated with a programming wand and the parameters altered depending on seizure frequency and side effects from the device. It may also be possible to taper anticonvulsant drugs if the patient achieves seizure freedom with the device.

Vagal nerve stimulation-related complications and side effects

The most common side effects of the procedure include infection, occurring in between 5% and 7% of patients. While it can be treated with oral antibiotics, one study showed that infection caused lead or generator removal in 1.5% of patients [16]. In this setting, reimplanation of the device is technically much more challenging.

Vocal cord paralysis occurs in around 1% of patients. Changes in phonation may improve following removal of the device itself, lead replacement, or changing the stimulation parameters. There is a concern about cardiac side effects, and while bradycardia and asystole have been reported intraoperatively in 0.1% of patients, this is possibly due to incorrect electrode placement, indirect cardiac nerve stimulation, accidental polarity reversal, or device malfunction. These cardiac effects are not usually seen postoperatively [20,21].

Other side effects, including hoarseness, throat pain, cough, vomiting, paresthesias, and, in children, dysphagia. Dyspnea remained commonly reported in 3.2% of patients but was classed as relatively mild by patients [16,22].

There is no increase in mortality with VNS compared with control groups, and sudden death in epilepsy rates appear to be lower in VNS than control, although this difference is not significant [23].

There was some concern that high-frequency stimulation could result in local tissue damage and also to the vagus nerve itself, but this has not been borne out in clinical experience. In particular, the self-sizing, helical nature of the coils of the electrodes minimizes damage of the nerve by the leads themselves. Likewise, the VNS system has a number of safeguards to limit the possible effects of the current on the nerve. For example, there is a "ramping up and down" feature for 2 s during each stimulation cycle, which allows for a gradual increase in stimulation rather than an immediate, maximum stimulation. Further, the voltage is limited by the VNS to 14 V, limiting the stimulation delivered to the nerve itself, and, if the patient finds the stimulation intolerable for whatever reason, the device can be deactivated by the use of a magnet placed over the generator for a period of time.

VNS can also improve mood and behavior, and has been suggested as a treatment for depression (Chapter 15) [24]. However, studies have also suggested that VNS can cause worsening of mood and behavior in patients with learning disabilities, but this is most likely due to improving seizure control rather than a direct effect of VNS itself.

Overall, therefore, side effects from VNS are minor, reversible and tend to improve with time, making it a well-tolerated treatment.

The device itself is safe in the presence of many radiofrequency transmissions and can be used near cellular phones and through airport security systems. However, it is not recommended for use with shortwave, microwave, or therapeutic ultrasound diathermy as this can cause heating of the stimulation system.

The manufacturer states that the device is also safe in head MRI, but a "transmit and receive" head coil should be used at 1.5 and 3 T field strengths. Inadvertent effects can include heating, particularly the stimulation electrodes, inadvertent magnet mode activation or resetting of the device, or direct damage to the device itself. The device should, however, be switched off with the output programmed to 0 for both the normal and magnetic settings, particularly if the pulse generator is implanted and the electrode inputs do not run parallel to the long axis of the body. Full body coil is not recommended, as this can cause undue heating of the leads and local tissue damage, and lengthy MRI sessions are also not advised. Likewise, phased-array head coils are not advisable, and even if the device is removed and the wire remains there could be effects as a consequence of the MRI. In these instances, it is recommended that the device manufacturer is consulted before undertaking any imaging studies using MRI [25].

Conclusions

There is evidence to suggest that VNS is an efficacious, palliative treatment for patients with medically refractory partial seizures who are not suitable for resective surgery. Its mechanism and exact indications remain controversial, with further work required to identify patients who are most likely to respond to the therapy, and also to understand its true mechanism of action. Despite this, VNS provides a non-pharmacological alternative to management of this complicated patient group.

Further reading

Englot, D.J., Chang, E.F. & Auguste, K.I. (2011) Vagus nerve stimulation for epilepsy: a meta-analysis of efficacy and predictors of response. *Journal of Neurosurgery*, **115** (6), 1248-1255.

Groves, D.A. & Brown, V.J. (2005) Vagal nerve stimulation: a review of its applications and potential mechanisms that mediate its clinical effects. *Neuroscience and Biobehavioral Reviews*, **29** (3), 493-500.

Heck, C., Helmers, S.L. & DeGiorgio, C.M. (2002) Vagus nerve stimulation therapy, epilepsy, and device parameters: scientific basis and recommendations for use. *Neurology*, **59** (6 Suppl. 4), S31-S37.

Schachter, S.C. (2002) Vagus nerve stimulation therapy summary: five years after FDA approval. *Neurology*, **59** (6 Suppl. 4), S15-S20.

Schachter, S.C. & Saper, C.B. (1998) Vagus nerve stimulation. *Epilepsia*, **39** (7), 677-686.

Tecoma, E.S. & Iragui, V.J. (2006) Vagus nerve stimulation use and effect in epilepsy: what have we learned? *Epilepsy & Behavior: E&B*, **8** (1), 127-136.

Uthman, B.M., Reichl, A.M., Dean, J.C. *et al.* (2004) Effectiveness of vagus nerve stimulation in epilepsy patients: a 12-year observation. *Neurology*, **63** (6), 1124-1126.

References

1 Hauser, W.A. & Kurland, L.T. (1975) The epidemiology of epilepsy in Rochester, Minnesota, 1935 through 1967. *Epilepsia*, **16** (1), 1-66.

2 Mattson, R.H., Cramer, J.A., Collins, J.F. *et al.* (1985) Comparison of carbamazepine, phenobarbital, phenytoin, and primidone in partial and secondarily generalized tonic-clonic seizures. *The New England Journal of Medicine*, **313** (3), 145-151.

3 Kwan, P. & Brodie, M.J. (2000) Early identification of refractory epilepsy. *The New England Journal of Medicine*, **342** (5), 314-319.

4 NICE [WWW document]. CG137 Epilepsy: NICE guideline URL http://guidance.nice.org.uk/CG137/NICEGuidance/pdf/English [accessed on 6 March 2013]

5 Lanska, D.J. (2002) J.L. Corning and vagal nerve stimulation for seizures in the 1880s. *Neurology*, **58** (3), 452-459.

6 Zabara, J. (1985) Time course of seizure control to brief, repetitive stimuli. *Epilepsia*, **26** (5), 518.

7 Penry, J.K. & Dean, J.C. (1990) Prevention of intractable partial seizures by intermittent vagal stimulation in humans: preliminary results. *Epilepsia*, **31** (Suppl. 2), S40-S43.

8 Aalbers, M., Vles, J., Klinkenberg, S. *et al.* (2011) Animal models for vagus nerve stimulation in epilepsy. *Experimental Neurology*, **230** (2), 167-175.

9   Paintal, A.S. (1973) Vagal sensory receptors and their reflex effects. *Physiological Reviews*, **53** (1), 159–227.

10 Asala, S.A. & Bower, A.J. (1986) An electron microscope study of vagus nerve composition in the ferret. *Anatomy and Embryology*, **175** (2), 247–253.

11 Fulwiler, C.E. & Saper, C.B. (1984) Subnuclear organization of the efferent connections of the parabrachial nucleus in the rat. *Brain Research*, **319** (3), 229–259.

12 Binnie, C.D. (2000) Vagus nerve stimulation for epilepsy: a review. *Seizure: The Journal of the British Epilepsy Association*, **9** (3), 161–169.

13 Nagarajan, L., Walsh, P., Gregory, P. *et al.* (2003) Respiratory pattern changes in sleep in children on vagal nerve stimulation for refractory epilepsy. *The Canadian Journal of Neurological Sciences*, **30** (3), 224–227.

14 Hsieh, T., Chen, M., McAfee, A. & Kifle, Y. (2008) Sleep-related breathing disorder in children with vagal nerve stimulators. *Pediatric Neurology*, **38** (2), 99–103.

15 Ben-Menachem, E., Manon-Espaillat, R., Ristanovic, R. *et al.* (1994) Vagus nerve stimulation for treatment of partial seizures: 1. A controlled study of effect on seizures. First International Vagus Nerve Stimulation Study Group. *Epilepsia*, **35** (3), 616–626.

16 Handforth, A., DeGiorgio, C.M., Schachter, S.C. *et al.* (1998) Vagus nerve stimulation therapy for partial-onset seizures: a randomized active-control trial. *Neurology*, **51** (1), 48–55.

17 DeGiorgio, C.M., Schachter, S.C., Handforth, A. *et al.* (2000) Prospective long-term study of vagus nerve stimulation for the treatment of refractory seizures. *Epilepsia*, **41** (9), 1195–1200.

18 Morris, G.L., 3rd & Mueller, W.M. (1999) Long-term treatment with vagus nerve stimulation in patients with refractory epilepsy. The Vagus Nerve Stimulation Study Group E01-E05. *Neurology*, **53** (8), 1731–1735.

19 Ben-Menachem, E. (2002) Vagus-nerve stimulation for the treatment of epilepsy. *Lancet Neurology*, **1** (8), 477–482.

20 Tatum, W.O.T., Moore, D.B., Stecker, M.M. *et al.* (1999) Ventricular asystole during vagus nerve stimulation for epilepsy in humans. *Neurology*, **52** (6), 1267–1269.

21 Asconape, J.J., Moore, D.D., Zipes, D.P. *et al.* (1999) Bradycardia and asystole with the use of vagus nerve stimulation for the treatment of epilepsy: a rare complication of intraoperative device testing. *Epilepsia*, **40** (10), 1452–1454.

22 Lundgren, J., Ekberg, O. & Olsson, R. (1998) Aspiration: a potential complication to vagus nerve stimulation. *Epilepsia*, **39** (9), 998–1000.

23 Annegers, J.F., Coan, S.P., Hauser, W.A. & Leestma, J. (2000) Epilepsy, vagal nerve stimulation by the NCP system, all-cause mortality, and sudden, unexpected, unexplained death. *Epilepsia*, **41** (5), 549–553.

24 Elger, G., Hoppe, C., Falkai P. *et al.* (2000) Vagus nerve stimulation is associated with mood improvements in epilepsy patients. *Epilepsy Research*, **42** (2-3), 203–210.

25 Cyberonics. [WWW document]. VNS Therapy® for Healthcare Professional. URL http://us.cyberonics.com/en/vns-therapy-for-epilepsy/healthcare-professionals [accessed on 6 March 2013].

Chapter 15

Vagal Nerve Stimulation in Treatment of Refractory Major Depression

Christine Matthews[1], Serenella Tolomeo[1], and Keith Matthews[2]

[1]University of Dundee, Dundee, UK
[2]Medical Research Institute, University of Dundee, Ninewells Hospital and Medical School, Dundee, UK

Introduction

Neurosurgical and neurostimulation interventions in psychiatry are consistent with contemporary biological approaches to the understanding of mental illness. Although earlier somatic approaches went "out of fashion" with the advent of late-twentieth-century neuropharmacological approaches to treatment, a recent resurgence in interest in such interventions has been driven by the continuing need for therapeutic alternatives. Vagal nerve stimulation (VNS) for treatment of refractory major depression (TRMD) has been explored as an alternative to electroconvulsive therapy and ablative neurosurgery.

VNS describes a procedure whereby the cervical portion of the left vagus nerve (VN) is stimulated electrically. This is achieved using the Neuro-Cybernetic Prosthesis (NCP™) system, manufactured by Cyberonics Inc., (Houston, TX). VNS was first approved for the treatment of pharmacoresistant epilepsy in 1994 (Europe) and in 1997 (USA). Subsequently, evidence emerged which suggested that patients showed simultaneous improvements in mood that were independent of any effects of VNS on epilepsy. One prospective study of 34 patients with epilepsy demonstrated a trend towards mood improvement in the 14 patients who received VNS therapy [1]. Along

Neurostimulation: Principles and Practice, First Edition. Edited by Sam Eljamel and Konstantin V. Slavin.
© 2013 John Wiley & Sons, Ltd. Published 2013 by John Wiley & Sons, Ltd.

with other observational evidence, this finding led Cyberonics to conduct a series of studies designed to examine the utility of VNS as a therapy in major depressive disorder (MDD).

The first Cyberonics-sponsored study (DO1) was an open-label feasibility trial of VNS which reported both acute (10 week) and longer-term outcomes for 59 participants [2,3,4]. Reports of a 30.5% response (15.3% remission) rate at 12 weeks, a 45% response rate (27% remission) at 12 months and a 43% response rate (21% remission) at 24-month follow-up were also published [2,5,6,7]. Although several other papers were published at this time, all observations were based on the original patient cohort of 59 as described by Sackheim *et al*. [5].

Following this, a larger-scale two-part study (DO2) was conducted. First, a randomized controlled trial of the acute effects of VNS which recruited a total of 235 participants, 210 with MDD and 25 with bipolar disorder. These patients received either masked active or sham VNS over 10 weeks. This study failed to demonstrate a clear difference between active and sham stimulation on the primary study end point. Subsequently, in a second phase of DO2, 205 members of the original cohort were evaluated at 12 months after either 9 or 12 months of open-label VNS. In this naturalistic study, VNS was well tolerated and a significant minority of patients (27%) appeared to improve, with 16% achieving remission. The characteristics of this cohort have also been described elsewhere [4,8,9,10,11,12,13,14].

A further observational study (DO4) compared outcomes for patients enrolled in the DO2 long-term study with a broadly comparable, VNS naïve, treatment-resistant population receiving "treatment as usual." Over 12 months, 27% of VNS patients showed significant improvement compared with 15% of the treatment-resistant population. Combined, these results prompted the US Food and Drug Administration to approve the use of VNS as an adjunctive treatment of refractory depression in 2005.

Subsequently an open-label multicenter study of VNS for chronic, medication-refractory MDD was conducted in Europe (DO3). Of the 74 subjects recruited, data for 70 participants were reported at 3 months, for 61 at 12 months, and for 49 at 2 years [15,16]. As in earlier studies, an apparent increase in benefit in response (42% or 25/59) and remission (22%) rates were seen over time. A number of other studies have also described this cohort [17,18,19,20,21,22].

We are aware of only one further study of VNS for the treatment of MDD. This was a phase IV clinical trial (D-21), registered as NCT 00305565, and it aimed to recruit 330 participants all of whom were diagnosed with either chronic or recurrent depression. The trial commenced in January 2006 and the last participant completed on February 2010. The protocol required that subjects have three successive exposures to a randomly assigned stimulation setting. One imaging publication has arisen from this study to date [23]. Further outcome data are awaited.

In addition to the literature already mentioned, where the main criteria for inclusion required a diagnosis of MDD with the patient experiencing a current and enduring depressive state, studies describing use in other conditions have also been reported in the literature [9,24,25]. Along with other material found, which falls into the category of review, correspondence, or critique, several case reports have also been published [26,27,28,29,30].

We have been able to identify a maximum of 450 individual patients in which VNS was used as a treatment for MDD. By contrast, in 2009 the UK National Institute for Health Care and Clinical Excellence (NICE) published a technology appraisal which concluded that a total of 1251 procedures had been conducted and reported. This appears to represent repeated counting of reported outcomes that were not different study participants. Summarizing the findings of 18 identified studies NICE went on to conclude that *the mechanism of action, predictors of outcome, differential responses and optimal stimulation parameters* remain unknown [30,31].

Referral criteria

With largely open-study data available on a cohort of fewer than 450 patients, VNS should continue to be considered as an experimental therapy. In delivering any experimental treatment it is essential that a participant is able to give informed consent. The individual must be empowered to make an autonomous, information-driven, voluntary decision about participation in therapy. Hence a meaningful and substantive exchange of information must take place prior to inclusion in any such therapeutic trial [32].

To facilitate this discussion, it is worth considering the manner in which VNS is portrayed in the literature. It has been suggested that VNS is both non-invasive and reversible. First, VNS cannot be described as non-invasive. In many respects, the Cyberonics NCP™ system is similar to an implanted cardiac pacemaker. A bipolar stimulating electrode is wrapped around the cervical portion of the left vagus nerve and connected subcutaneously to an implantable, programmable pulse generator located under the skin of the anterior left chest wall. This is achieved surgically in a procedure that usually takes about an hour. Therefore, while this procedure does not require *intracranial* surgery, it must still be considered invasive. Second, it is not clear how reversible a trial of VNS is. Once wrapped around the vagus nerve, the stimulating electrode cannot be removed without detailed micro-dissection. Indeed, it is common for extraction methods to leave the electrode in place when the remainder of the VNS system is explanted. In addition, VNS exerts effects by altering the activity of central neural pathways. The effect this has on neural function and possibly even structure remains unknown. It cannot be assumed that a cessation and withdrawal of stimulation will automatically lead to a reversal of effects and return to baseline functioning. Any prospective patient should be made aware of these issues. That said, of neurosurgical alternatives, VNS can be considered as *relatively* non-invasive and reversible.

It has been suggested that VNS may be more effective in patients with less treatment-resistant forms of depression, at least as defined by numbers of failed "adequate" antidepressant treatment trials [33]. This early study described a 50.0% response rate to VNS in patients failing trials of two or three antidepressants and a 29% response in those failing to respond to four to seven trials. Those failing seven or more previous antidepressant trials showed no response to VNS. Therefore, it was suggested that VNS therapy was more likely to be successful if used in patients with lower degrees of pharmacological treatment resistance. However, reflecting on the experimental nature of the therapy, the US FDA specified that VNS be reserved for use where patients had not experienced an adequate response to four or more antidepressant treatments.

For all patients considered for a trial of VNS, a detailed clinical assessment should be conducted. Structured clinical assessments should be used to confirm diagnosis and the presence of co-morbid conditions. Validated syndrome severity rating scales should be completed and a formalized assessment of the patient's ability to provide informed consent conducted. Crucially, VNS should not be considered the only treatment available at this stage. To facilitate consideration of all reasonable treatment options, the input during assessment by members of a multidisciplinary team whose members have complementary expertise is essential. Specifically, assessment of the adequacy of previous trials of psychological therapies should be performed, with recommendations for future management options. A robust assessment of the "adequacy" of ALL previous treatments (pharmacological, psychological, and ECT) must be conducted with a view to selecting the most appropriate therapeutic pathway for each patient and to provide alternatives for the patient to consider. These assessments and treatment discussions must be conducted *before* a surgeon is approached to consider implantation of a VNS system.

Assessment scales

All potential VNS patients should be assessed with respect to diagnosis, comorbidity, symptom burden, and functional impairment using standardized diagnostic instruments that generate diagnoses according to either ICD or DSM criteria, and rating scales should be used to describe baseline illness severity and level of functioning. Expanding on this, it is also helpful to make a rigorous assessment of quality of life and neurocognitive functioning in each patient. This should be completed at preoperative baseline, 12-month follow-up, and at longer-term (24–60 month) follow-up.

The following measures, or suitable alternatives, usually form the core of a comprehensive assessment battery for patients with refractory major depression who are to be treated with VNS:

Estimation of symptom burden

- Hamilton Depression Rating Scale, 17 item version (HDRS) [34]
- Montgomery-Asberg Depression Rating Scale (MADRS) [35]
- Clinical Global Impression (CGI) severity and improvement scales [36]
- Inventory of Depressive Symptoms (IDS$_{30}$-SR) self-report scale [37]
- Hospital Anxiety and Depression Scale (HADS) [38]
- Brief Symptom Inventory–Global Severity Index (BSI-GSI) [39]

Assessment of function

- Global Assessment of Function (GAF) [40]
- EuroQol 5-D (EQ-5D) [41]
- MOS SF-36 [42]

Neuropsychological assessment

- *Cambridge Neuropsychological Test Automated Battery (CANTAB)* [43]
  - Training and screening
    - Attention and memory
    - Non-strategic learning and memory
    - Sustained attention
    - Frontal/Executive tasks

Clinical neuropsychological testing

- National Adult Reading Test (NART) [44]
- Wechsler Memory Scale III (WMS-III) [45]
  - Information/orientation
  - List Learning
  - Paired associate learning
  - Logical Memory
  - Visual Reproduction
  - Digit Span
- Wechsler Adult Intelligence Scale-III (WAIS-III-R) [46]
  - Arithmetic
  - Comprehension
  - Block Design
  - Digit Symbol
  - Similarities
- Verbal Fluency Test/Controlled Oral Word Association Test [47]
- Stroop Test [48]
- Trial Making tests A&B [49]
- "6 elements" test from the Behavioural Assessment of the Dysexecutive Syndrome [50]

Rationale for vagal nerve stimulation in treatment of refractory major depression

While it is commonly understood to carry parasympathetic *efferent* fibers, as early as 1938 it was observed that the vagal nerve also conveyed sensory *afferent* projections to important brain areas by way of the nucleus tractus solitarius (NTS) [51]. It is now believed that approximately 80% of the fibers carried in the left vagus nerve are sensory afferents. They relay information on hunger, satiety, and pain to the nodose ganglion and the NTS in the medulla. From here, projections arise and communicate with brainstem median raphe and the locus coeruleus. These nuclei are dominant sources of serotonergic and noradrenergic innervation of limbic and neocortical structures. It is postulated that these fibers may mediate the therapeutic effects of VNS. Thus, application of direct electrical stimulation to the extracranial vagus nerve can result in modulation of the activity of structures such as the anterior cingulate, orbitofrontal cortex, hippocampus, and amygdala. These areas are widely considered to be important substrates in MDD [52]. VNS therapy has also been shown, using functional magnetic resonance imaging in MDD patients, to be associated with ventromedial prefrontal cortex deactivation and activation of the right insular cortex [53].

Programming parameters

As already mentioned, the VNS stimulator is normally implanted on the left side of the thorax. Stimulation of the right VN is avoided because of its potential effects on cardiac function [52]. Once implanted, the NCP™ VNS stimulator can be programmed using an external dose adjustment system or "wand." Controlled by a standard personal computer, electrode magnetic impulses from the wand regulate the output from the stimulating electrode. Data retrieval and simple diagnostic procedures can also be carried out in this way.

Programming parameters should be thought of in terms of *output current* (mA), *pulse* (µs), *frequency* (Hz) and *duration of stimulation*. As stimulation is applied intermittently, the duration is expressed as the percentage of time that the stimulator is ON relative to the time the stimulator is OFF. This is known as the *duty cycle*. Occasionally, the total *charge* (µC) delivered may also be reported. This can be calculated thus:

$$\text{charge (µC)} = \text{current (mA)} \times \text{pulse duration (µs)}.$$

Typically, although considerable variation has been reported in the literature, the following are often seen:

- current: range of 1.0-2.0 mA
- pulse duration: approximately 500 µs

- stimulation frequency: 20 and 30 Hz
- duty cycle: ON, 30 s; OFF, range 1.8–5 min.

Each of these parameters may be varied and adjusted to suit the individual using the external dose adjustment system described above. This allows the physician to calibrate the output of the VNS system at a level that is tailored to each individual patient's needs [54].

For patients who are struggling to tolerate the sensory effects of VNS, reduction in pulse width usually improves tolerability of stimulation. With standard settings (stimulator on for 30 s every 5 min), predicted battery life is between 5 and 10 years [52].

Monitoring, troubleshooting, complications, and side effects

Extensive experience with VNS for epilepsy suggests that adverse effects can be considered under two main headings: surgery related or VNS stimulation related.

The consequences of nerve damage and the range of stimulation-related adverse effects can be predicted by knowledge of the anatomy and functions of the left VN. There is a small risk of implant-related infection (around 1%), with a similarly low risk of physical damage to the left VN. The risk of nerve damage can be reduced if the stimulator is left inactive for 10–14 days after implantation. Around one-third of patients experience significant pain around the implant wound. Discomfort tends to recede with healing.

Generally, studies report mild adverse events with VNS. Commonly stimulation-related adverse effects include headache, neck, throat, pharynx, jaw and dental discomfort, hoarseness, alteration or loss of voice, cough, and difficulty in swallowing. These are however, frequently related to stimulation intensity. Consequently, by altering the current amplitude and pulse width, the severity of these effects can be ameliorated, or even abolished. Shorter pulse width usually permits increased current amplitude.

There is a general increase in tolerability of stimulation with the passage of time, but, in our experience, patients occasionally will describe an episodic, unexplained worsening of stimulation-related discomfort. It is rare for patients to have to use the supplied magnet to discontinue stimulation but many find reassurance in knowing that this facility is available. Some patients may describe stimulation settings as "tolerable" despite their obviously aversive quality. It is sometimes necessary to allow patients to test out the tolerability of stimulation settings for a period of hours before they depart from the clinic. Asking patients to drink a glass of water during a period of stimulation can provide useful confirmation that swallowing is not affected [52].

Serious adverse events have been reported in association with VNS therapy. Reports of manic mood switch, worsening depression and of suicide have been noted. In six acute phase treatment studies, three patients discontinued due to adverse events and three patients committed suicide

[2,5,15,18,19,55]. Another had a myocardial infarction, possibly related to stimulation [5]. The extent to which these reported effects were related to VNS is unclear. As suggested by Rush *et al.* [55] in 2005, adverse effect data should continue to be collated and analyzed as part of a systematic review strategy.

VNS does not appear to have negative effects on cognitive functioning and it has been reported that it may improve cognition in association with improvement in depression [16]. After 10 weeks of active VNS, Sackheim and colleagues reported that observed cognitive improvement may have indicated the reversal of neurocognitive deficits seen in depression [5].

Conclusion

VNS may represent a useful treatment option for patients with TRMD. However, the neurobiological rationale for this therapy has not been well established, it is moderately invasive, and involves a potentially irreversible procedure. The adverse effect profile is relatively favorable for most patients, but, there are some unresolved concerns about the possible association between VNS therapy and serious adverse events such as mood changes and suicide. Anyone receiving VNS for MDD should be closely followed up, with regular clinical review and recording of clinical status. Ongoing psychosocial support is also essential.

VNS for MDD should only be delivered by multidisciplinary clinical teams who have expertise in the management of such patients and who can provide the range of therapeutic options that are required by this population of patients. All patients should be kept under close clinical review and, where appropriate, clinical outcomes should be fully reported.

References

1 Harden, C.L., Pulver, M.C., Ravdin, L.D. *et al.* (2000) A pilot study of mood in epilepsy patients treated with vagus nerve stimulation. *Epilepsy & Behavior*, **1**, 93–99.

2 Rush, A.J., George, M.S., Sackheim, H.A. *et al.* (2000) Vagus nerve stimulation (VNS) for treatment-resistant depressions: a multicenter study. *Biological Psychiatry*, **47**, 276–286.

3 Nahas, Z., Marangell, L.B., Husain, M.M. *et al.* (2005) Two-year outcome of vagus nerve stimulation (VNS) for treatment of major depressive episodes. *The Journal of Clinical Psychiatry*, **66**, 1097–1014.

4 Sackheim, H.A., Brannan, S.K., Rush, A.J. *et al.* (2007) Durability of antidepressant response to vagus nerve stimulation (VNS). *International Journal of Neuropsychopharmacology*, **10**, 817–826.

5 Sackheim, H.A., Rush, A.J., George, M.S. *et al.* (2001) Vagus nerve stimulation (VNS) for treatment-resistant depression: efficacy, side effects, and predictors of outcome. *Neuropsychopharmacology*, **10**, 713–728.

6 Marangell, L.B., Martinez, M., Martinez, J.M. *et al.* (2005) Vagus nerve stimulation: a new tool for treating depression. *Primary Psychiatry*, **12**, 40–43.

7 Nahas, Z., Burns, C., Foust, M.J. *et al.* (2006) Vagus nerve stimulation (VNS) for depression: what do we know now and what should be done next? *Current Psychiatry Reports*, **8**, 445–451.

8 George, M.S., Rush, A.J., Marangell, L.B. *et al.* (2005) A one-year comparison of vagus nerve stimulation with treatment as usual for treatment-resistant depression. *Biological Psychiatry*, **58**, 364–373.

9 Nierenberg, A.A., Alpert, J.A., Gardner-Schuster, E.E. *et al.* (2008) Vagus nerve stimulation: 2-year outcomes for bipolar versus unipolar treatment-resistant depression. *Biological Psychiatry*, **64**, 455–460.

10 Burke, M.J. & Husain, M.M. (2006) Concomitant use of vagus nerve stimulation and electroconvulsive therapy for treatment-resistant depression. *The Journal of ECT*, **22**, 218–222.

11 Carpenter, L.L., Moreno, F.A., Kling, M.A. *et al.* (2004) Effect of vagus nerve stimulation on cerebrospinal fluid monoamine metabolites, norepinephrine, and gamma-aminobutyric acid concentrations in depressed patients. *Biological Psychiatry*, **56**, 418–426.

12 Carpenter, L.L., Bayat, L., Moreno, F. *et al.* (2008) Decreased cerebrospinal fluid concentrations of substance P in treatment-resistant depression and lack of alteration after acute adjunct vagus nerve stimulation therapy. *Psychiatry Research*, **157**, 123–129.

13 Conway, C.R., Sheline, Y.I., Chibnall, J.T. *et al.* (2006) Cerebral blood flow changes during vagus nerve stimulation for depression. *Psychiatry Research*, **146**, 179–184.

14 Pardo, J.V., Sheikh, S.A., Schwindt, G.C. *et al.* (2008) Chronic vagus nerve stimulation for treatment-resistant depression decreases resting ventromedial prefrontal glucose metabolism. *Neuroimage*, **42**, 879–889.

15 Schlaepfer, T.E., Frick, C., Zobel, A. *et al.* (2008) Vagus nerve stimulation for depression: efficacy and safety in a European study–Corrigendum. *Psychological Medicine*, **38** (5), 651–661.

16 Bajbouj, M., Merkl, A., Schlaepfer, T.E. *et al.* (2010) Two-year outcome of vagus nerve stimulation in treatment-resistant depression. *Journal of Clinical Psychopharmacology*, **30**, 273–281.

17 Bajbouj, M., Gallinat, J., Lang, U.E. *et al.* (2007) Motor cortex excitability after vagus nerve stimulation in major depression. *Journal of Clinical Psychopharmacology*, **27**, 156–159.

18 Neuhaus, A.H., Luborzewski, A., Rentzsch, J. *et al.* (2007) P300 is enhanced in responders to vagus nerve stimulation for treatment of major depressive disorder. *Journal of Affective Disorders*, **100**, 123–128.

19 O'Keane, V., Dinan, T.G., Scott, L. *et al.* (2005) Changes in hypothalamic-pituitary-adrenal axis measures after vagus nerve stimulation therapy in chronic depression. *Biological Psychiatry*, **58**, 963–968.

20 Corcoran, C.D., Thomas, P., Philips, J., & O'Keane, V. (2006) Vagus nerve stimulation in chronic treatment-resistant depression: preliminary findings of an open-label study. *The British Journal of Psychiatry: The Journal of Mental Science*, **189**, 282–283.

21 Zobel, A., Joe, A., Freymann, N. *et al.* (2005) Changes in regional cerebral blood flow by therapeutic vagus nerve stimulation in depression: an exploratory approach. *Psychiatry Research*, **139**, 165–179.

22 Kosel, M., Brockmann, H., Frick, C. *et al.* (2011) Chronic vagus nerve stimulation for treatment-resistant depression increases regional cerebral blood flow in the dorsolateral prefrontal cortex. *Psychiatry Research*, **191**, 153–159.

23 Conway, C.R., Sheline, Y.I., Chibnall, J.T. *et al.* (2011) Brain blood-flow change with acute vagus nerve stimulation in treatment-refractory major depressive disorder. *Brain Stimulation*, **1**, 227–228.

24 George, S., Ward, E., Ninan, P.T. *et al.* (2008) A pilot study of vagus nerve stimulation (VNS) for treatment-resistant anxiety disorders. *Brain Stimulation*, **1**, 112–121.

25 Christancho, P., Christancho, M.A., Baltuch, G.H. *et al.* (2011) Effectiveness and safety of vagus nerve stimulation for severe treatment-resistant major depression in clinical practice after FDA approval: outcomes at 1 year. *The Journal of Clinical Psychiatry*, **72**, 1376–1382.

26 Warnell, R.L. & Elahi, N. (2007) Introduction of vagus nerve stimulation into a maintenance electroconvulsive therapy regimen: a case study and cost analysis. *The Journal of ECT*, **23**, 114–119.

27 Husain, M.M., Stegman, D. & Trevino, K. (2005) Pregnancy and delivery while receiving vagus nerve stimulation for the treatment of major depression: a case report. *Annals of General Psychiatry*, **4**, 16.

28 Conway, R., Chibnall, T. & Tait, C. (2008) Vagus nerve stimulation for depression: a case of a broken lead, depression relapse, revision surgery, and restoration of patient response. *Brain Stimulation*, **1**, 227–228.

29 Critchley, H.D., Lewis, P.A., Orth, M. *et al.* (2007) Vagus nerve stimulation for treatment-resistant depression: behavioral and neural effects on encoding negative material. *Psychosomatic Medicine*, **69**, 17–22.

30 Daban, C., Martinez-Aran, A., Cruz, N. *et al.* (2008) Safety and efficacy of vagus nerve stimulation in treatment-resistant depression. A systematic review. *Journal of Affective Disorders*, **110**, 1–15.

31 National Institute for health and Clinical Excellence (December 2009) Vagus nerve stimulation for treatment resistant depression, IPG330.

32 Jotterand, F., McClintock, S.M., Alexander, A.A. *et al.* (2010) Ethics and informed consent of vagus nerve stimulation (VNS) for patients with treatment-resistant depression (TRD). *Neuroethics*, **3**, 13–22.

33 George, M.S., Sackheim, H.A., Rush, A.J. *et al.* (2000) Vagus nerve stimulation: a new tool for brain research and therapy. *Biological Psychiatry*, **47**, 287–295.

34 Hamilton, M. (1960) A rating scale for depression. *Journal of Neurology, Neurosurgery, and Psychiatry*, **23** (1), 56.

35 Montgomery, S.A. & Asberg, M. (1979) A new depression scale designed to be sensitive to change. *The British Journal of Psychiatry*, **134** (4), 382–389.

36 Guy, W. & Bonato, R. (1970) *CGI: Clinical Global Impressions: Manual for the ECDEU Assessment Battery 2*, revised edn. National Institute of Mental Health, Baltimore, MD.

37 Rush, A., Gullion, C.M., Basco, M.R. *et al.* (1996) The inventory of depressive symptomatology (IDS): psychometric properties. *Psychological Medicine*, **26** (3), 477–486.

38 Zigmond, A.S. & Snaith, R. (1983) The hospital anxiety and depression scale. *Acta Psychiatrica Scandinavica*, **67** (6), 361–370.

39 Derogatis, L.R. (1993) Brief Symptom Inventory: BSI; Administration, scoring, and procedures manual. Pearson.

40 Spitzer, R., Gibbon, M., Williams, J.B.W. *et al.* (1996) Global Assessment of Functioning (GAF) Scale. In: L.I. Sedere & B. Dickey (eds), *Outcome Assessment in Clinical Practice*. Baltimore: Williams and Wilkins, 76–78.

41 Sapin, C., Fantino, B., Nowicki, M.L. & Kind, P. (2004) Usefulness of EQ-5D in assessing health status in primary care patients with major depressive disorder. *Health and Quality of Life Outcomes*, **2** (1), 20.

42 McHorney, C.A., War, J.E., Jr, Lu, J.F.R. & Sherbourne, C.D. (1994) The MOS 36-item Short-Form Health Survey (SF 36): III. Tests of data quality, scaling assumptions, and reliability across diverse patient groups. *Medical Care*, **32**, 40–66.

43 Fray, P.J., Robbins, T.W. & Sahakian, B.J. (1996) Neuropsychiatric applications of CANTAB. *International Journal of Geriatric Psychiatry*.

44 Nelson, H. & Willison, J. (1991) *The Revised National Adult Reading Test-Test Manual*. NFER-Nelson, Windsor, ON.

45 Wechsler, D. (1997) *Wechsler Memory Scale (WMS-III)*. The Psychological Corporation, San Antonio, TX.

46 Wechsler, D. (1997) *Wechsler Adult Intelligence Scale (WAIS-III)*. The Psychological Corporation, San Antonio, TX.

47 Ruff, R., Light, R., Parker, S. & Levin, H. (1996) Benton controlled oral word association test: reliability and updated norms. *Archives of Clinical Neuropsychology*, **11** (4), 329–338.

48 Trenerry, M.R., Crosson, B., DeBoe, J. *et al.* (1989) *Stroop Neuropsychological Screening Test Manual*. Psychological Assessment Resources, Odessa, FL.

49 Reitan, R.M. & Wolfson, D. (1985) *The Halstead-Reitan Neuropsychological Test Battery: Theory and Clinical Interpretation*. Neuropsychology Press, Tucson, AZ.

50 Wilson, B.A., Evans, J.J., Emslie, H. *et al.* (1998) The development of an ecologically valid test for assessing patients with a dysexecutive syndrome. *Neuropsychological Rehabilitation*, **8** (3), 213–228.

51 Bailey, P. & Bremner, F. (1938) A sensory cortical representation of the vagal nerve. *Journal of Neurophysiology*, **1**, 405–412.

52 Matthews, K. & Eljamel, M.S. (2003) Vagus nerve stimulation and refractory depression: please can you switch me on doctor? *The British Journal of Psychiatry: The Journal of Mental Science*, **183**, 181–183.

53 Nahas, Z., Teneback, C., Chae, J.H. *et al.* (2007) Serial vagus nerve stimulation functional MRI in treatment resistant depression. *Neuropsychopharmacology*, **32**, 1649–1660.

54 Labiner, D.M. & Ahern, G.L. (2007) Vagus nerve stimulation therapy in depression and epilepsy: therapeutic parameter settings. *Acta Neurologica Scandinavica*, **115**, 23–33.

55 Rush, A.J., Marangell, L.B., Sackheim, H.A. *et al.* (2005) Vagus nerve stimulation for treatment-resistant depression: a randomized, controlled acute phase trial. *Biological Psychiatry*, **58**, 347–354.

Part 3
Motor Cortex Stimulation

Chapter 16

Mechanism of Action and Overview of Motor Cortex Stimulation Components

Sam Eljamel

University of Dundee, Ninewells Hospital and Medical School, Dundee, UK

Mechanism of action

The mechanism whereby motor cortex stimulation attenuates neuropathic pain remains unclear. However, whatever the precise actions underlying this effect, these are likely to be mediated by regional changes in brain synaptic activity, which should in turn be reflected by changes in regional cerebral blood flow (rCBF) [1]. rCBF changes can be tagged using functional imaging procedures, such as positron emission tomography (PET) in patients undergoing motor cortex stimulation (MCS).

Experimental studies in animals have demonstrated that electrical stimulation of the nervous system can exert strong inhibitory influences on pain transmission, thus prompting the use of neurostimulation strategies for the relief of chronic pain in humans. The neural targets of neurostimulation have been mostly the sensory pathways mediating transmission of non-noxious information (e.g., large afferent peripheral nerve fibers (peripheral nerve stimulation (PNS)), spinal dorsal columns or thalamic sensory nuclei) and to a lesser extent brainstem structures exerting antinociceptive influences, such as the periaqueductal or periventricular gray (PVG) (Chapter 11) matter [2,3]. Although stimulation of subcortical motor fibers was also shown to inhibit afferent transmission in the dorsal horn [4] and produce analgesic effects in man, the use of MCS for pain control was not reported and documented until the early 1990s [5]. Since then, MCS has been progressively introduced in functional neurosurgical procedures with the aim to treat chronic pain refractory to all pharmacological approaches [5,6,7]. Although

Neurostimulation: Principles and Practice, First Edition. Edited by Sam Eljamel and Konstantin V. Slavin.
© 2013 John Wiley & Sons, Ltd. Published 2013 by John Wiley & Sons, Ltd.

no randomized controlled study of MCS has been published yet and its use remains off-label, a number of case series covering more than 200 patients converge in indicating that 50-60% of patients with medically refractory neuropathic pain may benefit significantly from MCS, and that an even greater proportion would be willing to be operated again, should the same result be guaranteed [8].

Motor cortex stimulation components

MCS consists of components surgically implanted by the surgeon and external components to communicate with the implanted device.

The implantable components consist of:

(1) **An implantable pulse generator** (IPG) houses the battery and electronic components that regulate the stimulation parameters (Chapter 2).

(2) **A paddle lead implanted** in the epidural space over the motor cortex. These paddle leads were designed for spinal cord stimulation and have been used off label in MCS (Figure 16.1).

(3) **Lead extender** that connects each paddle lead to the IPG (Chapter 2). The IPG is implanted in the upper chest wall just below the collarbone (clavicle) on the side of the stimulated hemisphere or in the anterior abdominal wall using longer lead extenders. The junction between the deep brain stimulation (DBS) lead and the lead extender can be felt under the scalp often in the parietal region.

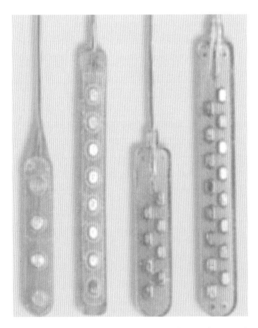

Figure 16.1 Paddle leads used in spinal cord stimulation and were used off label in motor cortex stimulation.

The non-implantable DBS components consist of:

(1) **Physician Programmer:** please see Chapter 2 for details.
(2) **Patient's controllers:** please see Chapter 2 for details.
(3) **Chargers for rechargeable IPGs:** please see Chapter 2 for details.

References

1 Sokoloff, L., Porter, A., Roland, P. *et al.* (1991) General discussion. In: C. Chadwick, J. Derek & J. Whelan (eds), *Exploring Brain Functional Anatomy with Positron Emission, Ciba Foundation Symposium*, pp. 43-56. Wiley and Sons, London.

2 Holsheimer, J. (1997) Effectiveness of spinal cord stimulation in the management of chronic pain: analysis of technical drawbacks and solutions. *Neurosurgery*, **40**, 990-999.

3 Wallace, B.A., Ashkan, K. & Benabid, A.L. (2004) Deep brain stimulation for the treatment of chronic, intractable pain. *Neurosurgery Clinics of North America*, **15**, 343-357.

4 Lindblom, U.F. & Ottosson, J.O. (1957) Influence of pyramidal stimulation upon the relay of coarse cutaneous afferents in the dorsal horn. *Acta Physiologica Scandinavica*, **38**, 309-318.

5 Tsubokawa, T., Katayama, Y., Yamamoto, T. *et al.* (1993) Chronic motor cortex stimulation in patients with thalamic pain. *Journal of Neurosurgery*, **78**, 393-401.

6 Mertens, P., Nuti, C., Sindou, M. *et al.* (1999) Precentral cortex stimulation for the treatment of central neuropathic pain: results of a prospective study in a 20-patient series. *Stereotactic and Functional Neurosurgery*, **73**, 122-125.

7 Meyerson, B.A., Lindblom, U., Linderoth, B. *et al.* (1993) Motor cortex stimulation as treatment of trigeminal neuropathic pain. *Acta Neurochirurgica. Supplementum*, **58**, 150-153.

8 Nuti, C., Peyron, R., Garcia-Larrea, L. *et al.* (2005) Motor cortex stimulation for refractory neuropathic pain: a study of long-term outcome and possible predictors of efficacy. *Pain*, **118**, 43-52.

Chapter 17
Motor Cortex Stimulation in Refractory Pain

Giovanni Broggi[1,2], Giuseppe Messina[1], Roberto Cordella[1], and Angelo Franzini[1]

[1]Fondazione Instituto Neurologico "Carlo Besta", Milan, Italy
[2]Ludes University, Lugano, Switzerland

Introduction

The connection between the motor cortex and pain circuits was suggested for the first time by Penfield, who observed some sensitive responses after stimulation of the motor cortex in a patient who had previously been submitted to removal of the postcentral cortex for treatment of epilepsy. Subsequently, White, Sweet, and Lende [1] performed postcentral corticectomies for the treatment of contralateral hemisomatic neuropathic pain, which were initially successful, and when pain relapsed they also removed the precentral gyrus, thus restoring the analgesic effect.

With the birth of neuromodulation era these initial encouraging results led to the concept of motor cortex stimulation for the treatment of different drug refractory painful conditions given the controversial results obtained with deep brain stimulation (DBS). The "gate control" theory of Melzack and Wall [2] was contradictory with such results, but this apparent contradiction paved the way for a deeper understanding of the complex pain-related circuits within the brain.

In 1991, Tsubokawa *et al.* [3] reported encouraging results of motor cortex stimulation (MCS) for the treatment of central deafferentation pain, hypothesizing that this procedure leads to an inhibition of thalamic burst discharges correlated with this condition.

Neurostimulation: Principles and Practice, First Edition. Edited by Sam Eljamel and Konstantin V. Slavin.
© 2013 John Wiley & Sons, Ltd. Published 2013 by John Wiley & Sons, Ltd.

Indications and referral criteria

The indications for MCS have expanded recently, and include drug refractory pain due to cerebral stroke, peripheral nerve injury pain, neuropathic facial pain, phantom limb pain, pain related to spinal cord injuries, and postherpetic neuralgia; several series report positive results in patients affected by these conditions. Usually the procedure is performed in patients who do not have medical contraindications to surgery, whose age is below 80 years, who present with a visual analogue scale (VAS) for pain of at least 50 and, who were refractory to three or more analgesic drugs administered for an "adequate" period of time [4]. Although these indications can vary from center to center, these general roles are used in most institutions.

Mechanisms of action

The exact mechanism of action of motor cortex stimulation in controlling painful symptoms is still unknown; nevertheless, several hypotheses have been made on the basis of anatomical and physiological knowledge, and the results of functional neuroimaging and electrophysiological studies. Some studies for example have demonstrated a normalization of the local somatosensory motor circuit [5] after MCS, suggesting the activation of intracortical non-nociceptive neurons of the primary sensory cortex; this control could be due to both orthodromic and antidromic pathways interconnecting motor and sensory cortices, and leading to activation of surrounding nociceptive inhibition in the sensory cortex. Canavero [6] hypothesized that the main mechanism is an increase in blood flow in the ipsilateral thalamus, which could reverse the disrupted oscillatory activity found in this structure in several painful conditions. Other authors have found that contralateral thalamus presented increased blood flow after successful MCS in patients with post-stroke pain [7]. Several functional imaging studies instead point to the role of different cortico-subcortical circuits involved in pain modulation; an increase in cerebral blood flow has also been observed in the anterior cingulate cortex, in the orbitofrontal cortex, posterior insula, and in the mediodorsal thalamus [8,9,10].

These structures are also involved in an affective dimension of pain perception; interestingly, the anterior cingulate cortex could influence the function of periacqueductal gray matter (PAG), which could in turn affect the activity state of the spinal cord's dorsal horn neurons [8,11]; and maybe through these pathways MCS could affect the endogenous opioid system as suggested by Maarrawi et al. [12].

Surgical procedure

The surgical procedure varies in different centers and also depends on preoperative examinations of choice; some centers report the use of functional magnetic resonance imaging (fMRI) for exact localization of the region within the motor cortex which represents the affected part of the body [8,13,14,15]; in this context, the use of fMRI is justified by the hypothesis that aberrant cortical plasticity occurs in patients with chronic pain [16,17]. MCS can be performed under general or local anesthesia, and consists of positioning of plate-shaped electrodes above the dura mater overlying the motor cortex, although some authors place them subdurally; in some centers the electrode is positioned parallel to the motor strip, and in others perpendicular to it, with the most anterior contacts located over the precentral gyrus. The procedure can be performed after localization of the precentral cortex based on neuroradiological anatomy, intraoperative somatosensory evoked potentials (SSEP), intraoperative stimulation, and, as stated previously, with the implementation of fMRI in the neuronavigation system (Figure 17.1).

Some authors perform MCS by sliding the plate electrode through a simple burr hole centered on the posterior portion of the previously localized precentral gyrus, whereas others perform a craniotomy [4]. Once positioned, the methods mentioned earlier can be used, permitting a refinement of the electrode position. For example, somatosensory evoked potentials are obtained after contralateral median nerve stimulation, and these are used to locate the contacts which allow the N20 phase reversal (P20) to be

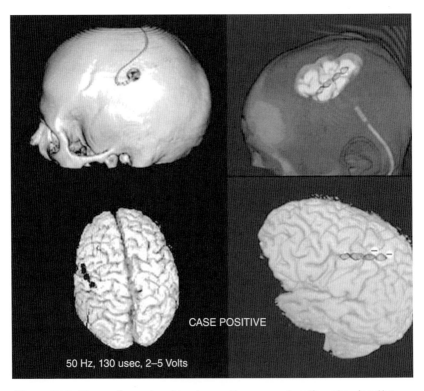

CASE POSITIVE

50 Hz, 130 usec, 2–5 Volts

Figure 17.1 Three-dimensional postoperative reconstruction showing the placement of the stimulation leads over the motor cortex.

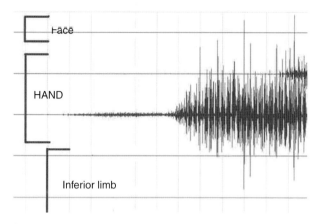

Figure 17.2 Intraoperative electromyograph (EMG) activity recorded from six muscles through monopolar pairs of electrodes placed under the skin. The sites were chosen to monitor the contralateral hemibody including the inferior limb, to assure selective EMG activation of the upper limb muscles.

recorded, also, various combinations of the contacts are used to stimulate the precentral gyrus until the affected region of the body presents motor-evoked potentials (Figure 17.2).

The lower limb representation lies in the medial surface of the hemisphere (anterior portion of the paracentral lobule), and positioning the electrode at this site may carry higher surgical risks and complications; for this reason, MCS is usually performed for facial or upper limb pain. Nonetheless, reports exist of placement of the electrode subdurally over the paracentral lobule, or epidurally very close to the sagittal sinus; in these cases, six out of 12 patients with lower limb pain improved by 40–50% [18].

Evidence base and results of motor cortex stimulation for pain

Recent reviews published by Fontaine *et al.* [18] and by Lima and Fregni [19] provide very useful data on overall clinical results of MCS used for chronic neuropathic pain; these reviews include several published articles which meet strict inclusion criteria, allowing for precise analysis of the results. The need for such systematic reviews of the literature stems out from the variability of the technique, indications, and evaluation scales of outcome; furthermore, only one randomized, controlled trial (RCT) for the determination of efficacy of MCS (in peripheral neuropathic pain) exists in the literature to date [4]. MCS is not unique in that the precise ideal indication is not well defined, mechanism of action is poorly understood and non-responders constitute significant number of those who received MCS therapy. Taking into account these potential confounding factors, the overall success rate of MCS for chronic pain in the Fontaine's study [18] (defined as a pain relief ≥40–50%)

was found in 55% of operated patients (in 45% of patients who have been followed-up for more than 1 year); the best results seem to have been achieved in patients with trigeminal neuropathic pain (68%). According to the meta-analysis by Lima and Fregni [19], 64% of patients presented a "positive" response to the treatment.

The most common reported adverse events include postoperative seizures (12%, with no report of subsequent chronic seizures), infections (5.7%), and hardware-related problems (5.1%).

As far as the RCT is concerned, the efficacy of the procedure was considered "good" or "satisfactory" in 60% of patients [4].

Conclusions

The lack of precise inclusion criteria, together with the imprecise understanding of the mechanisms of action of MCS makes it difficult to draw any kind of conclusions with regard to its efficacy, despite the review articles mentioned earlier. This is because objective data on the real (if any) rearrangements of cortical functionality due to possible aberrant cortical plasticity in any single case is very difficult to evaluate [20]. Assessment of the severity of pain, the underlying cause of painful symptoms, psychological issues, and the problem of the non-responder patients make this task even more difficult.

Nonetheless, encouraging results have been reported, and even though we still know very little about this intriguing neurosurgical procedure, ongoing refinements in functional neuroimaging, additional clinical studies, and increased experience in this therapeutic field will lead to an improvement in inclusion criteria and in the overall success rate.

References

1 Lende, R.A., Kirsch, W.M. & Druckman, R. (1971) Relief of facial pain after combined removal of precentral and postcentral cortex. *Journal of Neurosurgery* **34**, 537–543.

2 Melzack, R.A. & Wall, P.D. (1965) Pain mechanisms: a new theory. *Science* **150**, 971–979.

3 Tsubokawa, T., Katayama, Y., Yamamoto, T. *et al.* (1991) Chronic motor cortex stimulation for the treatment of central pain. *Acta Neurochirurgica. Supplementum,* **52**, 137–139.

4 Lefaucheur, J.P., Drouot, X., Cunin, P. *et al.* (2009) Motor cortex stimulation for the treatment of refractory peripheral neuropathic pain. *Brain: A Journal of Neurology,* **132** (Pt 6), 1463–1471.

5 Canavero, S. & Bonicalzi, V. (1995) Cortical stimulation for central pain. *Journal of Neurosurgery,* **83**, 1117.

6 Canavero, S. (1994) Dynamic reverberation. A unified mechanism for central and phantom pain. *Medical Hypotheses,* **42**, 203–207.

7 Saitoh, Y., Osaki, Y., Nishimura, H. *et al.* (2004) Increased regional cerebral blood flow in the contralateral thalamus after successful motor cortex stimulation in a patient with poststroke pain. *Journal of Neurosurgery*, **100**, 935-939.

8 Davis, K.D., Taub, E., Duffner, F. *et al.* (2000) Activation of the anterior cingulate cortex by thalamic stimulation in patients with chronic pain: a positron emission tomography study. *Journal of Neurosurgery*, **92**, 64-69.

9 Kishima, H., Saitoh, Y., Osaki, Y. *et al.* (2007) Motor cortex stimulation in patients with deafferentation pain: activation of the posterior insula and thalamus. *Journal of Neurosurgery*, **107**, 43-48.

10 Kupers, R.C., Gybels, J.M. & Gjedde, A. (2000) Positron emission tomography study of a chronic pain patient successfully treated with somatosensory thalamic stimulation. *Pain*, **87**, 295-302.

11 Garcia-Larrea, L. & Peyron, R. (2007) Motor cortex stimulation for neuropathic pain: from phenomenology to mechanisms. *Neuroimage*, **37** (Suppl. 1), S71-S79.

12 Maarrawi, J., Peyron, R., Mertens, P. *et al.* (2007) Motor cortex stimulation for pain control induces changes in the endogenous opioid system. *Neurology*, **69**, 827-834.

13 Esfahani, D.R., Pisansky, M.T., Dafer, R.M. & Anderson, D.E. (2011) Motor cortex stimulation: functional magnetic resonance imaging-localized treatment for three sources of intractable facial pain. *Journal of Neurosurgery*, **114** (1), 189-195.

14 Nguyen, J.P., Lefaucheur, J.P., Decq, P. *et al.* (1999) Chronic motor cortex stimulation in the treatment of central and neuropathic pain. Correlations between clinical, electrophysiological and anatomical data. *Pain*, **82**, 245-251.

15 Pirotte, B., Voordecker, P., Neugroschl, C. *et al.* (2005) Combination of functional magnetic resonance imaging-guided neuronavigation and intraoperative cortical brain mapping improves targeting of motor cortex stimulation in neuropathic pain. *Neurosurgery*, **56** (2 Suppl.), 344-359.

16 May, A. (2008) Chronic pain may change the structure of the brain. *Pain*, **137** (1), 7-15.

17 Buchner, H., Richrath, P., Grünholz, J. *et al.* (2000) Differential effects of pain and spatial attention on digit representation in the human primary somatosensory cortex. *Neuroreport*, **11**, 1289-1293.

18 Fontaine, D., Hamani, C. & Lozano, A. (2009) Efficacy and safety of motor cortex stimulation for chronic neuropathic pain: critical review of the literature. *Journal of Neurosurgery*, **110** (2), 251-256.

19 Lima, M.C. & Fregni, F. (2008) Motor cortex stimulation for chronic pain: systematic review and meta-analysis of the literature. *Neurology*, **70** (24), 2329-2337.

20 Messina, G., Cordella, R., Dones, I. *et al.* (2012) Improvement of secondary fixed dystonia of the upper limb after chronic extradural motor cortex stimulation in 10 patients: first reported series. *Neurosurgery*, **70** (5), 1169-1175.

Part 4
Spinal Cord Stimulation

Chapter 18

Mechanism of Action and Overview of Spinal Cord Stimulation Components

Sam Eljamel

University of Dundee, Ninewells Hospital and Medical School, Dundee, UK

Mechanism of action

The exact mechanism of spinal cord stimulation (SCS) is still unclear and it is likely to be multifactorial. One of the earliest explanations was the gate control theory of pain, described by Melzack and Wall [1]. It proposed that stimulation of large non-nociceptive myelinated nerve fibers of any peripheral nerve inhibited the activity of small nociceptive projections preventing (closing the gate) pain transmission in the dorsal horn of the spinal cord. This simplistic explanation did not stand the test of time, but the gate control theory laid down the foundation for further research to understand how SCS imparts its beneficial effects, why some patients respond while other do not, and why the effects of SCS may take some time to manifest whereas others fade away after initial good response. Research in this area highlighted several mechanisms by which SCS might work including:

(1) SCS leads to release of neurotransmitters in several areas along the pain pathways in the central nervous system. SCS is associated with GABA release in the periaqueductal gray (PAG) matter and dorsal horn (DH) of the spinal cord, and a decrease in the release of glutamate and aspartate. Experimental models of pain had also demonstrated that SCS leads to release of serotonin, glycine, adenosine, and norepinephrine (noradrenaline) and thus has an effect on descending pain pathways.

(2) SCS may also downregulate electric responses of peripheral nerves. Electrophysiological studies in rats with sciatic nerve injury showed SCS

Neurostimulation: Principles and Practice, First Edition. Edited by Sam Eljamel and Konstantin V. Slavin.
© 2013 John Wiley & Sons, Ltd. Published 2013 by John Wiley & Sons, Ltd.

inhibited hyperexcitability of wide dynamic range (WDR) neurons by lowering C-fiber response [2,3,4].

(3) SCS changes blood flow and metabolism in several areas of the nervous system. Positron emission tomography (PET) studies in patients with SCS for intractable neuropathic leg pain suggested SCS might modulate supraspinal neurons [5]. In these patients significant increases in regional cerebral blood flow were noted after SCS in the thalamus contralateral to the painful limb and in the associated bilateral parietal area that regulates pain threshold.

(4) SCS may also influence emotional responses to pain by activating anterior cingulate and prefrontal brain areas.

(5) SCS induces vasodilatation in the affected organ by reducing sympathetic activity and by antidromic vasodilatation via calcitonin gene-related peptides. This SCS-induced effect plays an important role in the mechanism by which SCS imparts beneficial effects in patients with intractable angina, complex regional pain syndrome (CRPS), and intractable peripheral ischemic pain and ulcers caused by peripheral vascular disease [6].

SCS does not seem to alter the levels or responses to opioids or opioid receptor-mediated analgesia, and the effects of SCS are not blocked by naloxone.

Spinal cord stimulation components

SCS consists of components surgically implanted and external components to communicate with the implanted device.

The implantable components consist of:

(1) **A pulse generator (IPG)** houses the battery and electronic components that regulate the stimulation parameters (Figure 18.1 gives some examples).

More than one company manufactures SCS systems and each IPG is able to drive current in a monopolar or bipolar fashion. The following parameters can be programmed: amplitude (Amp) measured in volts or milliamps, pulse width (PW) measured in microseconds, rate measured in hertz (Hz), and active contacts. For further details of commercially available systems please visit manufacturers' websites or contact your local neuromodulation providers.

(2) **An electrode implanted** into the epidural space at the level of the sweat spot of the spinal cord (SCS lead). There are several SCS leads on the market with two basic designs:

(a) **Percutaneous lead** that can be inserted under X-ray control and consists of four or more ring-type contacts, labeled from distal to proximal (Figure 18.2C,D,E).

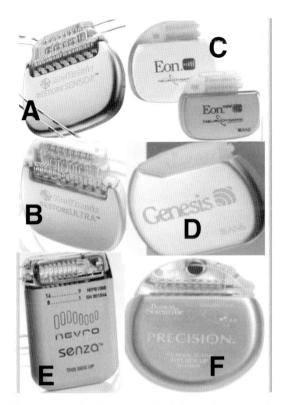

Figure 18.1 Photograph of different implantable pulse generators for spinal cord stimulation: Restore system (A, B) from Medtronic, EON (C) and Genesis (D) from St. Jude Medical, Precision (F) from Boston Scientific, and Senza (E) from Nevro.

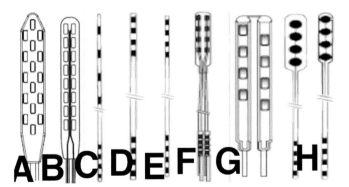

Figure 18.2 A–H, Examples of percutaneous and paddle spinal cord stimulation lead.

(b) **Paddle lead (surgical)** that needs laminotomy to implant and again consists of four or more flat contacts labeled numerically, these contacts can be arranged in a single row (Figure 18.2H), into left and right parallel rows (Figure 18.2B,E,G), or in more than two (up to five) rows (Figure 18.2A).

(3) **Lead extenders** that connect each lead to the IPG (Figure 18.3). Each SCS lead is compatible with multiple (but not all) lead extenders and each lead extender is compatible with multiple (but not all) IPGs. (Please check

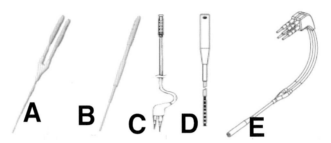

Figure 18.3 A–E, Examples of lead extenders.

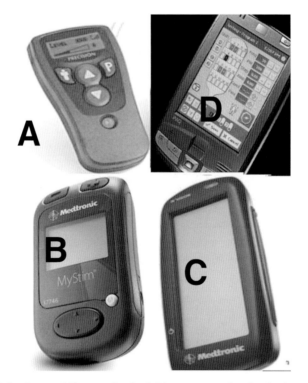

Figure 18.4 Some of the non-implantable components of spinal cord stimulation. A and B, Examples of patient controllers; C and D, examples of physician programmers.

the venders for the correct combinations and make sure that the equipment and implants are compatible; furthermore, some of the new devices will require adaptors for old leads and old lead extenders).

The IPG is usually implanted in the abdominal wall, chest wall, or the buttock area.

(4) **Lead fixators**

Each vender of a SCS system provides a lead fixator (anchor) to fix the SCS lead in place and prevent lead migration.

The non-implantable SCS components consist of:

(1) Physician programmer

The physician programmer consists of a programming wand, a hand-held device that interrogates and transmits programming parameters between a SCS therapy computer and the IPG, and a hand-held or laptop computer that allows the physician to interrogate and program the IPG (Figure 18.4C,D).

(2) Patient's controllers

Patient's controllers are hand-held devices used by patients to switch the IPGs on/off and to increase or decrease the stimulation within a range of parameters set by the physician (Figure 18.4A,B).

(3) Chargers for rechargeable IPGs

Some IPGs are rechargeable by patients.

References

1 Melzack, R. & Wall, P.D. (1965) Pain mechanisms: a new theory. *Science*, **150**, 971–979.

2 El-Khoury, C., Hawwa, M., Baliki, S.F. *et al.* (2002) Attenuation of neuropathic pain by segmental and supraspinal activation of the dorsal column system in awake rats. *Neuroscience*, **112**, 541–553.

3 Roberts, M.H.T. & Rees, H. (1994) Physiological basis of spinal cord stimulation. *Pain Reviews*, **1**, 184–198.

4 Wallin, J., Fiskå, A., Tjølsen, A. *et al.* (2003) Spinal cord stimulation inhibits long-term potentiation of spinal wide dynamic range neurons. *Brain Research*, **973**, 39–43.

5 Kishima, H., Saitoh, Y., Oshino, S. *et al.* (2010) Modulation of neuronal activity after spinal cord stimulation for neuropathic pain; H(2)^{15}O PET study. *Neuroimage*, **49**, 2564–2569.

6 Häbler, H.-J., Eschenfelder, S., Brinker, H. *et al.* (2000) Neurogenic vasoconstriction in the dorsal root ganglion may play a crucial role in sympathetic-afferent coupling after spinal nerve injury. In: M. Devor, M.C. Rowbotham & Z. Wiesenfeld-Hallin (eds), *Progress in Pain Research and Management*, pp. 661–667. IASP Press, Seattle.

Chapter 19

Spinal Cord Stimulation in Failed Back Surgery Syndrome

Gail Gillespie and Pravin Dandegaonkar

Ninewells Hospital and Medical School, Dundee, UK

Introduction

Failed back (or neck) surgery syndrome (FBSS/FNSS) refers to chronic back-leg or neck-arm pain that persists or recurs after spinal surgery for conditions such as disc herniation, lumbar stenosis, or spinal instability. It is also known as post-laminectomy syndrome or failed back syndrome and has considerable impact not only on individual patients but also on the healthcare system. The incidence of FBSS following lumbar spinal surgery is commonly quoted as being in the range of 10% to 40%. The etiology of FBSS is often multifactorial. These factors may occur in the preoperative, intraoperative, and postoperative periods (Table 19.1). Despite advances in surgical technology, the rates of FBSS have remained the same; instead, the number of patients suffering from FBSS has increased with increasing rates of spinal surgery [1]. Comparing international data, the rates of spine surgery in the USA are double that of other developed countries such as Australia, Canada, and Finland and five times greater than the UK. The impact of FBSS on an individual's quality of life and functional status are considerable and more disabling than other common chronic pain conditions like arthritis. These findings emphasize the importance of identifying strategies to prevent the development of FBSS and to effectively manage established FBSS.

The treatment of FBSS is often interdisciplinary and based on individual patient's needs. Apart from conventional medical management, invasive treatment options including spinal cord stimulation (SCS) are important treatment considerations. Indeed, FBSS remains the commonest indication for implantation of SCS in the USA, and it has been recommended by both

Neurostimulation: Principles and Practice, First Edition. Edited by Sam Eljamel and Konstantin V. Slavin.
© 2013 John Wiley & Sons, Ltd. Published 2013 by John Wiley & Sons, Ltd.

Table 19.1 Etiology of failed back surgery syndrome (adapted from [17])

Preoperative factors
Revision surgery
Poor candidate or wrong choice of surgery
Patient with psychosocial risk factors (anxiety, depression, litigation, work compensation)

Intraoperative factors
Incorrect level of surgery
Poor surgical technique (e.g., inadequate lateral recess decompression)

Postoperative factors
Epidural fibrosis
Surgical complications (e.g., nerve injury, infection, and hematoma)
Progressive disease (e.g., recent disc herniation)
New spinal instability

the National Institute for Health and Clinical Excellence (NICE) and the British Pain Society in UK [2,3].

Since the first case that demonstrated the safety and utility of SCS in 1967 in a patient with cancer pain, there has been a steady growth in the literature proving its efficacy, as well as ongoing refinements in device technology. SCS has also been used in the management of pain in patients with complex regional pain syndrome (CRPS), peripheral vascular disease, refractory angina, and post-amputation pain (mostly for the stump pain, but also for some cases of phantom limb pain). The use of SCS in patients with FBSS not only improves pain and quality of life but also reduces opioid consumption and allows some patients to return to work. It may also result in significant cost savings over time and associated adverse effects are often minor.

Rationale for spinal cord stimulation

Since the times of the Ancient Greeks, who used torpedo fish to treat the pain of gout arthritis, much like electric therapies to treat disease, SCS continues to undergo evolution. There have been multiple theories put forward to explain the neuromodulation mechanisms through which SCS provides analgesia in various painful conditions. The persistence or recurrence of pain in the back and/or legs following spinal surgery leads to the diagnosis of FBSS. Neuropathic pain that results from damage to the somatosensory system is often present in the form of shooting, stabbing, and burning sensations with radiation into buttocks and legs. Additionally, axial pain localized to the lower back contributes to a variable degree. Although individuals with predominantly neuropathic extremity pain are still widely acknowledged to be the best candidates for this treatment, recent advances in SCS technology such as dual electrodes have improved analgesic coverage in patients with axial spine pain [4].

One of the earliest theories that inspired the introduction of SCS was the gate control theory of pain, described by Melzack and Wall [5]. According to this theory, the stimulation of large non-nociceptive myelinated fibers (A beta fibers) of the peripheral nerves inhibited the activity of small nociceptive projections (A delta and C fibers), causing inhibition of pain transmission in the dorsal horn of the spinal cord. This theory has since been shown to be incomplete, and now there is increasing evidence to suggest that SCS causes pain modulation by supraspinal activity via the posterior columns of the spinal cord. SCS is associated with GABA release in the periaqueductal gray matter and dorsal horn, and a decrease in the release of glutamate and aspartate. Experimental evidence has also shown that SCS changes neurochemistry by releasing serotonin, glycine, adenosine, and norepinephrine (noradrenaline) and thus has an effect on descending pain pathways. Electrophysiological studies in rats with sciatic nerve injury showed that SCS inhibited hyperexcitability of wide dynamic range (WDR) neurons by lowering C-fiber response [6].

Positron emission tomography (PET) studies in patients with SCS for intractable neuropathic leg pain suggest that SCS also modulates supraspinal neurons [7]. In these patients significant increases in regional cerebral blood flow were noted after SCS, both in the thalamus contralateral to the painful limb and in the associated bilateral parietal area that regulates the pain threshold. SCS also influenced emotional response to pain by activating anterior cingulate cortex and prefrontal areas. There appears to be no relationship between SCS and endogenous opioid receptor-mediated analgesia, however, as the effects of SCS are not blocked by naloxone.

SCS-induced vasodilatation, by a reduction in sympathetic activity and antidromic vasodilatation via calcitonin gene-related peptide, plays an important role in patients with CRPS and ischemia.

Referral criteria for spinal cord stimulation

Once the diagnosis of FBSS is established, the overall goal for patient selection for SCS is to choose those patients most likely to experience therapeutic success while reducing the likelihood of complications and adverse events. A careful assessment by a multidisciplinary team, and discussion of the patient's expectations and goals, will help identify appropriate candidates for SCS. Neuropathic buttock and leg pain can often be successfully treated, but the associated back pain which may have both nociceptive and neuropathic component can be difficult to treat with this technique. However, advances in device technology and variable lead configurations have evolved to meet this need.

SCS is not only an invasive procedure but is also associated with significant cost implications. With growing emphasis on evidence-based medical practice and current healthcare system where every technology is scrutinized for cost effectiveness, it would be useful to know the subgroup of patients with FBSS who are most likely to benefit from the use of SCS.

Table 19.2 Referral criteria for spinal cord stimulation therapy in patients with failed back surgery syndrome

> **Pain features**
> Chronic, intractable pain for more than 6 months.
> Inadequate relief from more conventional treatments.
> Pain is predominantly radicular or radiating rather than axial in distribution.
> Pain is neuropathic rather than nociceptive in nature.
> Pain has objective evidence of pathology and distribution is consistent on examination and diagnostic imaging.
> The pain is adequately relieved during an SCS screening trial.
>
> **Patient characteristics**
> 18 years of age or older
> Non-pregnant
> Patient can properly operate the system
> Patient understands therapy risks
> Patients with no evident unresolved major psychiatric comorbidity
> No secondary gain issues or active substance abuse disorder
> Initial or further surgical intervention not indicated
> No contraindications to therapy
> Therapy and function goals have been established
> Patients have preserved posterior column function

We consider that patients with FBSS who fulfill the following criteria (Table 19.2) may benefit from SCS treatment and can be used by healthcare professionals, including referrers or clinicians involved in SCS.

Assessment of a patient with failed back surgery syndrome for spinal cord stimulation

A patient with FBSS, as with any other chronic pain syndrome, should undergo detailed assessment, including clinical history, examination, and necessary investigations. This initial evaluation will be essential in order to

(1) establish the nature and cause of pain leading to FBBS diagnosis;
(2) assist in excluding serious pathology or need for surgical referral;
(3) ensure appropriate conventional and multidisciplinary management is followed;
(4) identify suitable candidates for SCS trial and implantation.

General principles

History

Details of postoperative symptoms including pain should be obtained and its comparison with preoperative findings will provide an insight into possible causes. It is useful to identify if the pain is mainly nociceptive or neuropathic in nature as treatment options differ. Predominantly radicular pain may be due to epidural fibrosis, recurrent disc herniation, or incomplete decompression. Careful review of surgical reports, medical notes, and previous imaging can identify events such as incorrect initial diagnosis or surgery at the wrong level. Early surgical referral should be sought in the presence of any red flags (e.g., new focal neurological deficit, cauda equina symptoms, malignancy, or inflammatory processes) or if there are any surgically correctable factors (e.g., misplaced pedicle screw or misplaced graft). A validated numeric rating scale or visual analogue scale can help to decide pain intensity and follow the patient's progress, but an indication of degree of functional limitation should also be explored. The pain treatment history and comorbid medical history should be obtained as this may influence choice of treatments.

Significant psychosocial stressors are known to play an important role in chronic pain conditions (FBSS being no exception); hence, specific inquiry must attempt to identify the presence of anxiety, depression, inadequacy of coping mechanisms, substance misuse, or issues of secondary gain (e.g., ongoing litigation, worker's compensation). This is especially important if secondary surgery is planned, as the failure rates for revision surgery is higher in these patients. Such psychological evaluation is vital in the consideration of suitability of a patient for SCS as it provides valuable information to guide patient selection. It identifies the small percentage of patients who might benefit from psychological treatment prior to SCS or in whom SCS might be complicated by psychosocial factors. Medicare in the USA and other private insurers requires a psychological evaluation before SCS implantation while expert consensus reveals a high likelihood of a favorable outcome in properly selected patients.

Examination

The physical examination is similar to any initial patient evaluation but will be largely directed by the patient's history. Standard tests of posture, range of motion, signs of nerve root tension, and neurological examination are performed. The interpretation of non-organic physical findings such as pain behavior is controversial, but recent research has suggested their presence as indicative of psychological distress [8]. The examination should exclude other possible common causes of back and or leg pain involving facet joints, sacroiliac joints, disc problems, scar tenderness, spinal canal stenosis, and vascular insufficiency.

Investigations

The choice of investigations is guided to an extent by the findings on history and clinical examination. The commonly performed imaging studies to establish FBSS diagnosis include plain radiographs, magnetic resonance imaging (MRI) or computed tomography (CT) myelogram and provide information about a patient's postsurgical anatomy and whether anatomical goals of surgery were met or not. Laboratory tests to identify markers of infection are indicated in the presence of constitutional symptoms such as fever or rigors. Electromyograms or nerve conduction studies are rarely performed but may be helpful to assess the severity and location of nerve injury, to evaluate extraspinal neural compression or rule out peripheral neuropathy.

Plain radiographs can evaluate surgical site, changes in alignment, degenerative changes, and degree of resection of posterior segments. Flexion-extension views are useful in a patient who has had fusion surgery and may show the presence of instability, pars defect, or deformity.

MRI provides most useful information in investigating the cause of symptoms. Gadolinium-enhanced MRI can differentiate between postoperative epidural fibrosis (scar tissue) and residual or recurrent disc herniation. Although epidural fibrosis is common following spinal surgery, studies have demonstrated that the severity of scar tissue correlates with recurrence of pain [9] and patients with extensive scarring were 3.2 times more likely to experience recurrent radicular pain than patients with less scarring [10]. The presence of gadolinium enhancement in the intervertebral disc and vertebral bodies may indicate postoperative infection. MRI can also reveal information such as stenosis in the lateral recess and neural foramina or discitis. Recent MRI of the anticipated SCS implantation site (e.g., thoracic spine for FBSS) prior to SCS trial is advised to exclude canal stenosis that may be critically exacerbated by implantation of SCS hardware into an already narrowed epidural canal. This is particularly important for patients being considered for paddle lead implantation.

CT myelography is indicated in patients where MRI is contraindicated (e.g., patients with pacemakers) or MRI scans are degraded by hardware artifact. CT myelogram is useful in demonstrating compression of neural structures by bony elements and is also able to evaluate dynamic problems like instability or impingement.

Contraindications for spinal cord stimulation

- Absolute contraindications
  - significant cognitive deficits
  - nerve compression amenable to surgery and causing serious neurological deficit
  - gross instability at risk of progression
  - uncontrolled coagulopathy, immunosuppression, or other condition associated with an unacceptable surgical risk (e.g., local or systemic infection).
- Relative contraindications
  - local or systemic infection
  - presence of a demand pacemaker or defibrillator
  - presence of a major comorbid chronic pain syndrome

- anticoagulant or antiplatelet therapy
- occupational risk (e.g., employment requires climbing ladders or operating certain machinery or vehicles or working in hyperbaric conditions)
- unrealistic expectations of SCS
- failure to engage (e.g., frequent non-attendance at clinic appointments).

The generic steps of a pathway for a patient who undergoes SCS therapy include: (1) multidisciplinary assessment, (2) patient educational session, (3) screening trial, (4) permanent implantation, and (5) long-term care.

Multidisciplinary assessment ideally involves all members of the SCS team: surgeon, pain physician, physiotherapist, specialist nurse practitioner, and clinical psychologist. This provides a global patient assessment to establish diagnosis, assess functional impact of pain, assess suitability for SCS, and undertake psychosocial evaluation. Based on this assessment the patient can be deemed appropriate and ready for SCS, or unsuitable with plans for alternative pain management options. A subgroup of patients may need further input such as psychological intervention or education about pain management strategies prior to embarking upon SCS.

Educational sessions can be conducted with a patient and/or caregivers 2-4 weeks in advance of the planned SCS screening trial. The clinician or neuromodulation specialist nurse practitioner will be able to discuss and establish realistic goals and expectations with the patient. It is important for a patient to understand that with SCS there would be around 50% chance of achieving 50% or more pain relief (i.e., not "pain free") and where possible this may reflect in some improvement in daily life activities. Furthermore, it is imperative that pain self-management is reinforced including pacing, graded exercise, flare-up planning, and goal setting. The patient should be educated in the whole process involved, including familiarity with relevant devices and their usage. This can be supported by providing them with written and audiovisual information or by arranging discussion meetings with other patients who have such devices implanted. This step serves the idea of informed decision-making process on behalf of the patient and ensures that the patient has the vital pain self-management strategies in place prior to moving to the next steps. Further appointments to focus on any shortfalls may be necessary before proceeding to trial.

The outcome of the SCS trial is to provide valuable information about the potential technical and clinical success of SCS. It involves insertion of a percutaneous epidural lead (Chapter 18) under local anesthesia. For a patient with FBSS with radicular leg pain, the lead is placed under fluoroscopic guidance in the epidural space at the T8-T10 level and adjusted to provide optimum lower limb coverage. On stimulation, using the external pulse generator, the patient will experience a tingling sensation (paresthesia), and it is important to cover the area of pain with this paresthesia. The paresthesia must be comfortable; there should be no motor stimulation or undue paresthesia outside the painful area. This often needs adjusting of electrode position, trying different stimulation settings, electrode combinations or overlapping programs. The area of epidural space should be mapped so as to guide the position of the surgical electrode for future permanent implantation (assuming the SCS trial is successful). A patient typically undergoes 3–7 days of screening trial and is labeled successful if there are gains of 50% or more of pain relief with SCS use, and no major side effects. The trial period also gives an idea whether the patient experiences any improvement in daily activities and allows estimation of battery usage to assist choice of IPG for permanent implant. When a trial is unsuccessful, the lead is removed and alternative options to manage the pain should be considered. For successful cases permanent implantation is planned.

Full implantation involves either internalization of the percutaneous trial lead (especially in areas where neurosurgical support is unavailable) or removal of the trial lead at the end of the trial, then at a future date, a paddle is surgically placed (Chapter 18) via laminotomy/laminectomy. In both cases this is then connected to the IPG implanted in the lateral abdominal wall (preferred) or upper buttock (e.g., if pregnancy planned in future). The procedure is carried out under intravenous sedation or general anesthesia, depending on technique, patient, and operator choices. Meticulous aseptic and surgical technique is paramount to minimize complications. On-table test stimulation is recommended to establish the paresthesia/pain overlap. After routine postoperative check-up, system integrity is checked with the physician programmer before the patient's discharge. The patient should return for wound check-up, staple/suture removal in 7–14 days' time, and SCS programming adjustments if required.

Subsequent long-term care will involve routine follow-up visits, depending on local resources and patient requirements. We taper follow-up visits from one at 6 weeks, followed by reviews at 3 and 6 months each and every year thereafter. Patients should be aware of precautions required with the SCS system (e.g., possible switch off where electromagnetic fields are encountered and avoiding activities that may put strain on the implanted system) and have access to SCS services in case of an emergency or for troubleshooting problems.

Evidence for use of spinal cord stimulation in patients with failed back surgery syndrome

The outcome of SCS therapy can be based on patient-reported outcome measures and procedure-related technical outcomes. The primary outcome measure in patients with FBSS is pain relief, with an efficacious result deemed to be 50% or more pain reduction. Commonly used secondary outcome measures include medications use, changes in quality of life and daily function, patient satisfaction, impact on comorbid symptoms (depression, neurological functions), and return to work. Frey et al. [11] in a recent systematic review on SCS for patients with FBSS highlighted the paucity and heterogeneity of available literature. The evidence to date comes from two good-quality randomized controlled trials (RCTs) and a few observational studies. As SCS in its current and most widely used form is associated with paresthesia, blinding in clinical trials is not feasible.

In 2005, North et al. [4] undertook a prospective RCT (crossover study) in which 50 FBSS patients were randomized to SCS or repeat spinal surgery. At a mean follow-up of 2.9 years, 47% of SCS patients reported 50% or more pain relief compared with just 12% of patients with reoperation ($p < 0.01$) while use of opioid analgesics was significantly less in SCS patients ($p < 0.025$). Patients initially randomized to SCS were significantly less likely to cross over than were those randomized to reoperation (5 of 24 vs 14 of 26). None of the patients who crossed over from SCS to surgery achieved success while six of 14 who crossed over to SCS found benefit. The two groups did not show significant differences in work status and daily activities.

An international multicenter RCT (PROCESS study) randomized 100 patients with predominant radicular leg pain secondary to FBSS to either conventional medical management (CMM) alone or CMM plus SCS. Patients randomized to SCS plus CMM achieved significantly greater pain relief, after 6 months (48% vs 9%) and 12 months (48% vs 18%). The SCS group also showed a significantly greater improvement in function, health-related quality of life, and better patient satisfaction than CMM alone, while no dif-ference was noted with regards to return to work. Findings from other observational studies also showed positive results for both short- and long-term pain relief.

A concern with SCS therapy has been the high initial acquisition cost associated with the equipment. In 2008, NICE (UK) published guidance [2] with regard to cost effectiveness of SCS following systematic reviews and technology assessment. By using a decision analytic model (which compared the cost of treating FBSS with SCS versus CMM and reoperation), it was predicted that SCS would produce added quality-adjusted life years at a cost the UK health service would be willing to pay. The evidence from various cost-effectiveness analyses suggests that SCS is associated with high initial cost but lowers the total cost of care of patients with neuropathic pain compared with alternative treatments such as CMM or reoperation for FBSS.

Complications

Although SCS provides a relatively safe, reversible, and non-destructive option to treat pain, it is not free of complications. Prospective studies assessing adverse events are rare; therefore, the data for complication rates are extrapolated. The complications can be broadly categorized into biologi-cal complications, and equipment-related and other complications.

Overall complication rates are reported at about 34–38%, with lead migra-tion being the most common [12,13]. The majority of these complications are minor and amenable to simple treatments or minor surgical procedures. Potential life-threatening problems are very rare. Kumar et al. [14] reported that biological complications are common within the first 3 months after SCS implantation while equipment-related complications continue to occur for the first 2 years following implantation.

Reported incidence of equipment-related complications varies from 6% to 34.3%. Cameron [13], based on his literature review involving 2972 patients, reported the complication rate of lead migration as 13.2%; lead fracture as 9.1%; hardware malfunction as 2.9%; and unwanted stimulation as 2.4%. Lead migration occurs more commonly with percutaneous leads than surgically implanted paddle leads and occurs more often in the cervical region than thoracolumbar area. Lead migration can be minimized by properly fixing the leads to ligaments or by using of anchors, whereas minimum use of connectors and the use of strain relief loops can reduce lead fractures. The problems of generator or battery failure are also reported. With improvement in technology, using programs and training patients in techniques to preserve battery life, or implanting generators with rechargeable batteries, these problems can largely be addressed.

Biological complications include superficial infection at the generator or connector site, or at the site of lumbar incision (approximately 5%), but infections in the spinal canal are very rare. *Staphylococcus aureus* is the most commonly reported organism, followed by *Pseudomonas*. Infections can be reduced by stringent aseptic techniques, and administration of prophylactic antibiotics. In suspected infections, superficial infections often respond to treatment with oral or intravenous antibiotics; however, revision or explantation is required in those cases that fail to respond. Rarely, seroma (non-infectious serosanguinous fluid collection) can form at the site of the pulse generator and may require treatment such as pressure application, needle aspiration, or incision and drainage. The commonest neurological complication associated with percutaneous SCS implantation is inadvertent dural puncture with an estimated incidence of 6–11%. Previous surgery at the site of needle placement, spinal stenosis, calcified ligamentum flavum, patient movement, and obesity are the risk factors for dural puncture. Postdural puncture headache may respond well to conservative treatment including adequate hydration and caffeine. The role of epidural blood patch as a treatment strategy remains controversial in the presence of SCS because of the risk of infection and fear of displacement of leads. The alternative option may necessitate removal of leads prior to carrying this out in refractory cases. Alò *et al.* [15] found that the most common reason for explantation was pain at the site of the pulse generator. More serious neurological complications such as epidural hematoma or direct injury to the spinal cord or nerve roots by the needle or electrodes are very rare. Rare case reports of paraplegia, seizures, quadriparesis, bladder disturbances, and increased neuropathic pain have been reported. A recent summary of SCS implantation techniques indicated that the incidence of serious neurological deficit is higher than previously thought [16].

Other complications mainly involve failure to stimulate the painful area or painful thoracic dermatome stimulation due to an unsatisfactory electrode position. Changes in patient posture may affect SCS stimulation, but newer

IPGs can be programmed to sense and allow adjustments in stimulation in such situations. A small percentage of patients find paresthesias associated with SCS more unpleasant than their pain (this should be evident at the trial stage) while some patients may lose SCS effectiveness over longer periods (also known as system tolerance), presumably due to plasticity of pain pathways and/or local epidural fibrosis [14].

Future developments

Neurostimulation including SCS has undergone significant advancements to minimize equipment-related complications, provide better analgesic coverage, and to meet demands associated with expanding application of neurostimulation, coupled with competitiveness of neuromodulation industry. Improvements include better, less fracture-prone leads; better anchor designs to mitigate lead migration; and smaller, more powerful rechargeable IPGs. There is much interest in expanding the MRI compatibility of SCS. A new generation of leads will permit more contacts per lead (up to 64 plus) from the current 16 contacts, providing physicians greater versatility to treat complex pain syndromes. With the development of percutaneous multilead systems and approval for use of percutaneous delivery tools, the need for invasive surgical laminotomy will be reduced. Preliminary results from Europe about the use of high-frequency SCS (HFSCS; 5000-10 000 Hz), which provides paresthesia-free analgesia, showed that it could achieve pain relief of back and leg pain in patients who are refractory to conventional SCS. Further work is required to understand the mechanism of HFSCS and its clinical efficacy in the long term.

Conclusions

FBSS remains a challenging clinical entity for both patients and clinicians. Patients with FBSS will benefit from multidisciplinary management including the use of SCS. The available literature suggests that SCS therapy is efficacious in terms of improved pain scores, improved quality of life, and, despite initial high cost, has proven to be cost effective in the long term. With advancements in SCS systems to improve safety and efficacy, SCS has now moved ahead of long-term opioid therapy, spinal reoperations, and intrathecal drug delivery and should be considered alongside conventional medical treatment for patients with FBSS.

Further reading

Chan, C.W. & Peng, P. (2011) *Review article: failed back surgery syndrome. Pain Medicine*, **12**, 577-606.

North, R.B. & Shipley, J. (2007) *Practice parameters for the use of spinal cord stimulation in the treatment of neuropathic pain. Pain Medicine*, **8** (S4), S200-S275.

References

1 Talbot, L. (2003) *Failed back surgery syndrome. British Medical Journal (Clinical Research Edition),* **327**, 985-987.
2 National Institute for Health and Clinical Excellence (NICE) technology appraisal guidance 159 (2008) *Spinal cord stimulation for chronic pain of neuropathic or ischaemic origin.* URL http://www.nice.org.uk/nicemedia/live/12082/42367/42367.pdf [accessed 18 July 2012].
3 The British Pain Society (2009) *Spinal cord stimulation for the management of pain: recommendations for best clinical practice (consensus document).* URL http://www.britishpainsociety.org/book_scs_main.pdf [accessed 12 June 2012].
4 North, R.B., Kidd, D.H., Olin, J. *et al.* (2005) *Spinal cord stimulation for axial low back pain: a prospective, controlled trial comparing dual with single percutaneous electrodes. Spine,* **30**, 1412-1418.
5 Melzack, R.A. & Wall, P.D. (1965) *Pain mechanisms: a new theory. Science,* **150**, 971-979.
6 Wallin, J., Fiskå, A., Tjølsen, A. *et al.* (2003) *Spinal cord stimulation inhibits long-term potentiation of spinal wide dynamic range neurons. Brain Research,* **973**, 39-43.
7 Kishima, H., Saitoh, Y., Oshino, S. *et al.* (2010) *Modulation of neuronal activity after spinal cord stimulation for neuropathic pain; H(2)^{15}O PET study. Neuroimage,* **49**, 2564-2569.
8 Carleton, R.N., Kachur, S.S., Abrams, M.P. & Asmundson, G.J. (2009) *Waddell's symptoms as indicators of psychological distress, perceived disability, and treatment outcome. Journal of Occupational Rehabilitation,* **19**, 41-48.
9 Bosscher, H.A. & Heavner, J.E. (2010) *Incidence and severity of epidural fibrosis after back surgery: an endoscopic study. Pain Practice,* **10**, 18-24.
10 Ross, J.S., Robertson, J.T., Frederickson, R.C. *et al.* (1996) *Association between peridural scar and recurrent radicular pain after lumbar discectomy: magnetic resonance evaluation. Neurosurgery,* **38**, 855-863.
11 Frey, M.E., Manchikanti, L., Benyamin, R.M. *et al.* (2009) *Spinal cord stimulation for patients with failed back surgery syndrome: a systematic review. Pain Physician,* **12**, 379-397.
12 Turner, J.A., Loeser, J.D., Deyo, R.A. & Sanders, S.B. (2004) *Spinal cord stimulation for patients with failed back surgery syndrome or complex regional pain syndrome: a systematic review of effectiveness and complications. Pain,* **108**, 137-147.
13 Cameron, T. (2004) *Safety and efficacy of spinal cord stimulation for the treatment of chronic pain: a 20-year literature review. Journal of Neurosurgery,* **100**, 254-267.
14 Kumar, K., Wilson, J.R., Taylor, R.S., Gupta, S. (2006) *Complications of spinal cord stimulation, suggestions to improve outcome, and financial impact. Journal of Neurosurgery. Spine,* **5**, 191-203.
15 Alò, K.M., Redko, V. & Charnov, J. (2002) *Four-year follow-up of dual electrode spinal cord stimulation for chronic pain. Neuromodulation,* **5**, 79-88.
16 Levy, R., Henderson, J., Slavin, K. *et al.* (2012) *Incidence and avoidance of neurologic complications with paddle type spinal cord stimulation leads. Neuromodulation,* **14**, 412-422.
17 Chan, C.W. & Peng, P. (2011) *Review article: failed back surgery syndrome. Pain Medicine,* **12**, 577-606.

Chapter 20

Spinal Cord Stimulation in Complex Regional Pain Syndrome

Eduardo Goellner[1] and Konstantin V. Slavin[2]

[1]Hospital Mãe de Deus, Porto Alegre/RS, Brazil
[2]University of Illinois at Chicago, Chicago, Illinois, USA

Introduction

Complex regional pain syndrome (CRPS) is a neuropathic disorder characterized by continuous pain that is disproportionate to the inciting event and is associated with trophic changes and functional impairment. The pathophysiology is not completely understood, but it is probably related to the development of abnormal arc reflexes involving structures of the peripheral, the sympathetic, and the central nervous systems. The origin of the symptoms may follow minor traumas or immobilization of the extremities, classified as CRPS I (formerly known as reflex sympathetic dystrophy (RSD)), or be present after an evident lesion of a nerve trunk, called CRPS II (formerly known as causalgia) [1].

The annual incidence for CRPS calculated in a population-based study was 26.2 per 100 000 persons [2]. It is estimated that around 20% of the cases will become chronic, and, to date, there is no single effective treatment for these patients. The result is frequently a devastating condition, leading to personal and social losses.

A multidisciplinary approach with physiotherapy, medications, and psychotherapy is the most appropriate management to reduce the pain and restore function of the affected limb. The final goal should be an improvement in the patient's quality of life [3].

Spinal cord stimulation (SCS) has been shown to be effective in different chronic pain conditions and is an important option for the treatment of refractory CRPS [3,4].

Neurostimulation: Principles and Practice, First Edition. Edited by Sam Eljamel and Konstantin V. Slavin.
© 2013 John Wiley & Sons, Ltd. Published 2013 by John Wiley & Sons, Ltd.

History and taxonomy

Despite isolated historical descriptions of patients with pain after peripheral nerve traumas, Weir Mitchell was the first to describe the signs and symptoms of the syndrome that is known today as CRPS. In his monograph *Gunshot Wounds and other Injuries of Nerves*, published in 1864 with the contribution of Morehouse and Keen, he presented his experience with soldiers from the Union Armies wounded during the American Civil War. The term causalgia (from the Greek *kausis*—burning, and *algos*—pain) appeared just 3 years later in Mitchell's article *United States Sanitary Commission Memoirs* in 1867, after the suggestion of Robley Dunglison [5].

The term *reflex sympathetic dystrophy* (RSD) was first introduced by James Evans in 1846. Wolff, in 1883, used this term to describe trophic changes in the extremities of patients with infectious arthritis. Later in 1900, Sudeck published his classic description of burning pain, edema, cutaneous lesions, and bone atrophy after trauma in extremities without clear nervous lesion [6].

Roberts, in 1986 [7], hypothesized the neuronal mechanism of RSD and causalgia studying the response of treatment with sympathetic block, using the expression *sympathetically maintained pain* (SMP). Similarly, the term sympathetically independent pain (SIP) can be used for patients who do not improve with sympathetic block.

Different names were used to define signs and symptoms that in essence were very similar or had the same origin. This lack of uniformity brought some confusion to the diagnosis, making a comparison between diverse treatments difficult. Responding to this issue, the International Association for the Study of Pain (IASP) created in 1994 the term *complex regional pain syndrome* (CRPS) [8].

At that time, neuropathic continuous pain following trauma or immobilization of the limbs that is disproportionate to the inciting event and associated with vasomotor or trophic changes with the tendency to develop motor and functional limitations were grouped into a single syndrome. The etiology of the pain is the reason for the division into CRPS I, formerly known as RSD, where there is no clear lesion to the nerve, and CRPS II, previously called causalgia, where there is an evident lesion of the nerve trunk. Also, the terms SMP and SIP can be used in both situations.

Diagnosis and classification

According to recommendations of the IASP, the diagnosis of CRPS is made based on its signs and symptoms. These include pain, sensory alterations, and vasomotor changes. Since adoption of the IASP classification improves the sensitivity of the diagnosis of RSD and causalgia, the treatment of this condition may be started earlier. However, this approach has a tendency to overestimate the disease. The recent inclusion of motor and trophic changes

Table 20.1 Diagnostic criteria for complex regional pain syndrome (CRPS) based on the modified International Association for the Study of Pain classification

Diagnostic criteria for CRPS
1 Continuing pain that is disproportionate to any inciting event
2 Presence of at least one symptom in three of the four categories a sensory: reports of hyperesthesia and/or allodynia b vasomotor: reports of temperature asymmetry and/or skin color changes and/or skin color asymmetry c edema and/or sweating changes and/or sweating asymmetry d motor/trophic: reports of decreased range of motion, and/or motor dysfunction (weakness, tremor, dystonia), and/or trophic changes (hair, nails, skin)
3 The presence of at least one sign in two or more of the four categories a sensory: evidence of hyperalgesia (to pinprick) and/or allodynia (to light touch and/or temperature sensation and/or deep somatic pressure and/or joint movement) b vasomotor: evidence of temperature asymmetry (>1°C) and/or skin color changes and/or asymmetry c sudomotor/edema: evidence of edema and/or sweating changes and/or sweating asymmetry d motor/trophic: evidence of decreased range of motion and/or motor dysfunction (weakness, tremor, dystonia) and/or trophic changes (hair, nails, skin)
4 No other diagnosis that could explain the sings or symptoms

improves the specificity of the diagnosis, and a new classification was proposed by a consensus of pain specialists in Budapest in 2007 [9] (Table 20.1).

CRPS can occur in any part of the body, most commonly in extremities after trauma (fracture, contusion, surgery), or immobilization, and less often after venous puncture, infection, myocardial infarction, venous thrombosis, or without obvious cause.

- Pain has disproportionate intensity and duration to the inciting event. Usually it is located in the affected segment of the limb, but later it may spread to the entire arm or leg, other side (mirror), or less frequently to an unrelated body part. The characteristics and descriptions of CRPS pain may vary from burning, shock-like or stabbing, continuous or intermittent, superficial or deep.
- The patient may report all kinds of sensory alterations: paresthesia, hypoesthesia, or anesthesia, hyperesthesia, or allodynia. Similar to pain, these complaints are usually limited to the affected limb but may also spread to other areas.
- The features of CRPS include not only subjective but also objective findings. There are autonomic dysfunctions with changes in skin temperature (hot or cold), color (purple, red, or pale), sweating (hyper or hypohidrosis), and edema. These features may change over time. They also may be constantly present or be elicited by tactile stimuli or emotions.

- Trophic abnormalities may be present in any structure: skin (thin or thick), hair, and nails (fragile with growth delay), tendon (retraction), and bone (osteoporosis or erosion).
- Motor changes that may be encountered in CRPS patients are weakness, muscle spasm, tremor, or dystonia. In the beginning, the patient has a tendency not to use the affected part trying to prevent pain. Later, it may translate into a stable change in position from atrophy or cutaneous, tendinous or bone deformities.
- Psychiatric problems such as depression and sleep disorder are not considered diagnostic features of CRPS, but they are frequently present in chronic CRPS patients. It is important to consider that most of the time mood disorders are not the cause but the consequence of this complex neuropathic condition.

CRPS can also be classified into three different stages: acute, dystrophic, and atrophic.

- The first, acute phase is characterized by pain, and neurovegetative and sensitivity changes. These early symptoms usually start around 0–3 months after the inciting event, but may occur years after the hypothetic cause of the syndrome. The inflammatory response in this phase has an important role in the pathophysiology of the disease.
- Second, the dystrophic stage includes all of the initial signs and symptoms plus the trophic and motor alterations. It usually occurs between the third and ninth months.
- Finally, the atrophic phase is marked by the progression of the cutaneous, tendinous, and bone abnormalities, leading to deformities and functional limitations of the extremities.

Complementary examinations, such as X-rays, computed tomography, magnetic resonance imaging or scintigraphy, do not make the diagnosis of CRPS but help to define the current stage of the disease and its impact on the structural tissues.

Criteria for referral to spinal cord stimulation

CRPS I

Generally, any patient with chronic CRPS I with poor disease control after conservative treatments is a candidate to receive neuromodulation therapy. The final indication is based on response to the trial with SCS and the absence of contraindications. Patients with poor cognitive function, unrealistic expectations, or any clinical disease that elevates the risks of surgical intervention should not be treated with SCS. Patients with depression or history of drug abuse are not excluded from the trial, but the disease must be under control.

Patients with good response to sympathetic block have higher chances of a positive response to SCS trial and subsequent long-term SCS treatment [10], but SIP patients could also benefit from stimulators and a stimulation trial is therefore indicated. Cervical and lumbar SCS showed the same pain relief scores [11]. Patients under 40 years of age and those who started SCS therapy within 1 year of the syndrome onset tend to have better outcomes [12]. Brush-evoked allodynia may be a negative predictive factor [13].

CRPS II

The obvious lesion of the nerve trunk in the pathophysiology of CRPS II makes the open exploration of the affected structure the first surgical option after failed non-invasive modalities. The goal is to release the nerve from compression or adhesions, eliminating the noxious event. In case of complete transection, repair with nerve graft could be an alternative. SCS is reserved for those patients who continue experiencing pain after exploratory surgery, and a trial of SCS is indicated once the failure of exploratory surgery is documented.

Rationale of spinal cord stimulation in complex regional pain syndrome

The real pathophysiology of CRPS is still unknown. The initial mechanism seems to be related to local inflammatory process, common to any noxious event. The maintenance of this circle, either from extrinsic or intrinsic factors, would unbalance the regulation of neurotransmissions, leading to pain and vasomotor symptoms. This could happen at the level of the peripheral nerve, the dorsal root ganglion, or the central nervous system.

The increased sympathetic tone may be involved in this process. Peripherally, the reason would be the upregulation of adrenergic receptor α-1 or the decreased reuptake of presynaptic epinephrine (adrenaline) [14,15]. In central pathways, abnormal firing in the dorsal horn would spread to the intermediolateral column. The result is vasoconstriction, ischemia, and disproportional pain. These theories help explain the benefit of sympathetic block in some patients, but they do not provide an answer for the unresponsiveness of others.

Another theory postulates that the persistent activation of unmyelinated C nociceptors and Aδ fibers would sensitize the neurons from the laminae V of the dorsal column, which in turn could be activated by different afferent input. Low-threshold mechanoceptors via myelinated A fibers could produce allodynia by light touch. Continuous pain and vasomotor changes could result from activation of the sympathetic fibers [7]. The abnormal neurotransmission is mediated by substance P, glutamate, and N-methyl-D-aspartate.

The effect of SCS on CRPS could be the suppression of the abnormal hyperexcitability of high-threshold nociceptive spinothalamic neurons in the dorsal horn. Also, the activation of interneurons at or nearby the substantia gelatinosa could consequently inhibit the deeper laminae III–V in the dorsal column. Excitation of supraspinal sites such as pretectal nucleus that produces analgesia by inhibiting nociceptive dorsal horn neurons is also possible. Finally, it is known that the release of adenosine, 5-hydroxytryptamine, and glycine, and the activation of gamma aminobutyric acid receptors by SCS would decrease the excitation at dorsal column [16,17,18].

Therefore, there is erratic communication among peripheral, central, and sympathetic systems that is abnormally maintained. The role of any therapeutic approach, including SCS, is to interrupt this vicious cycle, restoring the normal synaptic pathways.

Assessment methods

The treatment of CRPS is multidisciplinary and starts with physiotherapy, medications, and psychotherapy. It should be started as soon as the symptoms begin or the diagnosis of the syndrome is raised, after excluding other causes. The aim is to improve the quality of life and to delay or stop the progression of the disease. Unfortunately, around 20% of patients become chronic and need other adjunctive therapy.

Sympathetic block is an option according to the response to diagnostic test. Sympathectomy, an option from in the past, is no longer routinely performed because of the great number of potential side effects, at times irreversible.

Once conservative treatment fails or control of the symptoms is not adequate, a trial with SCS should be offered. There is no consensus regarding the right time to start SCS. If it is done at an early stage, surgical intervention may be over indicated, as natural (spontaneous) improvement may still take place. If it is performed too late, patients who could have some relief with SCS will suffer unnecessarily. It is not clear that SCS would prevent CRPS from spreading to other areas, but patients who start this treatment earlier tend to have better outcomes [19]. We believe that after 6 months of uncontrolled disease, patients in whom symptoms are stable or deteriorating should be considered for SCS trial, and patients in whom symptoms are improving, surgical intervention could be postponed.

The trial is performed with the electrode inserted in the spinal epidural space, covering the dermatome with symptoms. We prefer to use a permanent electrode fixed to the fascia through a small incision that is connected to a temporary extension lead attached to an external generator. This decreases the chances of different coverage later with the permanent device. Patients are tested for a minimum of 7 days. The trial is considered positive if there is a reduction in pain using a visual analog scale (VAS) of at least 50%. The external connection is then cut and the patient undergoes placement of an IPG that is connected to the epidural electrode already in place (Figure 20.1).

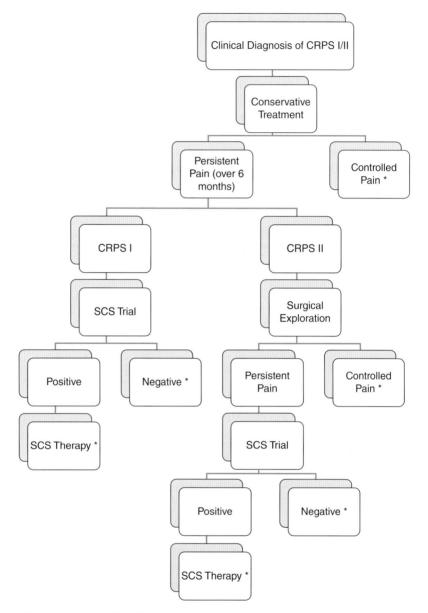

Figure 20.1 Algorithm for the treatment of complex regional pain syndrome with spinal cord stimulation.

Evidence for spinal cord stimulation in complex regional pain syndrome

SCS has been used for the treatment of CRPS for decades in thousands of patients. Many articles have been written supporting the use of SCS, most of them case report series and retrospective studies. A systematic review of the literature performed by Taylor et al. [20] reported pain relief of at least 50% over a median follow-up of 33 months in 67% of the patients with CRPS I and II treated with SCS therapy (95% CI: 51–84%). They did not find predictor factors for pain relief. There is level A evidence for CRPS type I patients and level D for type II, supporting treatment with SCS. Taking into consideration economical aspects, SCS also seems to be cost-effective in the long-term compared with conventional treatment alone [21].

Nevertheless, there is only one randomized clinical trial comparing SCS plus physical therapy versus physical therapy alone (high level of evidence). At 2 years of follow-up, Kemler et al. [22] showed higher pain reduction and global perceived effect and improved health-related quality of life with the SCS group. But at 5 years of follow-up there was no significant difference between groups. Interestingly, 90% of the SCS patients answered that they had positively responded to the treatment, and 95% would repeat the treatment for the same results [22]. Sears et al. [23] also found differences analyzing positive responses, suggesting that the VAS may not be the ideal measuring tool in the evaluation of long-term outcomes.

Another prospective study showing good results with SCS for CRPS I was conducted by Harke et al. [24] with a follow-up period of 35.6 ± 21 months. Deep pain and allodynia were reduced from 10 to 0–2 on the VAS ($p < 0.01$), functional status and quality of life improved, and pain medication was reduced. The selection of only SIP patients could have skewed the study towards better outcomes.

The indication of SCS in early stages of CRPS was questioned by van Eijs et al. [25] because of the good prognosis of patients in the first year of the disease. This question was addressed earlier in this chapter.

Most common programming settings

The stimulation begins with programming settings and contacts that best covers the affected area and with no side effects. The frequency is adjusted from 70 to 120 Hz, and the pulse width from 100 to 500 μs. Because there is a lack of literature discussing programming settings for CRPS, it is reasonable to begin with low parameters to prevent battery drainage. The amplitude is set as low as possible to produce paresthesia. Impedance is checked regularly. The pattern of stimulation is modified according to clinical outcome. It is important to wait at least several weeks before making further adjustments.

Potential side effects and complications

The potential side effects and complications related to SCS and CRPS are very similar to other indications in a range of 30–63%. Hardware-related problems are disconnection, fracture, or migration of the lead (most common), and pulse generator malfunction. Technical complications include post-spinal puncture headache, hematoma, pain over the implant, and skin erosion. Most of these side effects can be solved with revision surgery, reprogramming the device, or simply by turning it off. The infection rate varies from 0.4% to 4%. The risks of permanent neurological sequela are extremely low.

Conclusions

SCS has been used for the treatment of refractory pain syndromes for decades with a broad spectrum of applications. CRPS is a devastating condition that has a chance of becoming chronic in 20% of patients. When conservative multimodality treatment fails, SCS trial should be considered in order to reduce pain and improve the patient's quality of life. Its indications are based on case series and few prospective studies, but the efficacy of SCS for CRPS has been consistently shown in all published reports. Further research focused on the pathophysiology of this neuropathic disorder and randomized controlled trials on the longevity of SCS for CRPS are needed.

References

1 Stanton-Hicks, M., Janig, W., Hassenbusch, S. *et al.* (1995) Reflex sympathetic dystrophy: changing concepts and taxonomy. *Pain*, **63** (1), 127-133.

2 de Mos, M., de Bruijn, A.G., Huygen, F.J. *et al.* (2007) The incidence of complex regional pain syndrome: a population-based study. *Pain*, **129** (1-2), 12-20.

3 Kemler, M.A., Barendse, G.A., van Kleef, M. *et al.* (2000) Spinal cord stimulation in patients with chronic reflex sympathetic dystrophy. *The New England Journal of Medicine*, **343** (9), 618-624.

4 Kemler, M.A., Barendse, G.A., Van Kleef, M. *et al.* (1999) Electrical spinal cord stimulation in reflex sympathetic dystrophy: retrospective analysis of 23 patients. *Journal of Neurosurgery*, **90** (1 Suppl.), 79-83.

5 Richards, R.L. (1967) The term 'causalgia'. *Medical History*, **11** (1), 97-99.

6 Sudeck, P. (1900) Über die akute entzuü ndliche Knochenatrophie. *Archiv fur Klinische Chirurgie*, **62**, 147-156.

7 Roberts, W.J. (1986) A hypothesis on the physiological basis for causalgia and related pains. *Pain*, **24** (3), 297-311.

8 Merskey, H. & Bogduk, N. (1994) Classifications of chronic pain: description of chronic pain syndromes and definition of pain terms. In: H. Merskey & N. Bogduk (eds), *Report by the International Association for the Study of Pain Task Force on Taxonomy*, pp. 209-214 IASP Press, Seattle.

9 Harden, R.N., Bruehl, S., Stanton-Hicks, M. & Wilson, P.R. (2007) Proposed new diagnostic criteria for complex regional pain syndrome. *Pain Medicine (Malden, Mass.)*, **8** (4), 326-331.

10 Hord, E.D., Cohen, S.P., Cosgrove, G.R. *et al.* (2003) The predictive value of sympathetic block for the success of spinal cord stimulation. *Neurosurgery*, **53** (3), 626-632; discussion 32-33.

11 Forouzanfar, T., Kemler, M.A., Weber, W.E. *et al.* (2004) Spinal cord stimulation in complex regional pain syndrome: cervical and lumbar devices are comparably effective. *British Journal of Anaesthesia*, **92** (3), 348–353.

12 Kumar, K., Rizvi, S. & Bnurs, S.B. (2011) Spinal cord stimulation is effective in management of complex regional pain syndrome I: fact or fiction. *Neurosurgery*, **69** (3), 566–578; discussion 5578–5580.

13 van Eijs, F., Smits, H., Geurts, J.W. *et al.* (2010) Brush-evoked allodynia predicts outcome of spinal cord stimulation in complex regional pain syndrome type 1. *European Journal of Pain*, **14** (2), 164–169.

14 Arnold, J.M., Teasell, R.W., MacLeod, A.P. *et al.* (1993) Increased venous alpha-adrenoceptor responsiveness in patients with reflex sympathetic dystrophy. *Annals of Internal Medicine*, **118** (8), 619–621.

15 Raja, S.N., Treede, R.D., Davis, K.D. & Campbell, J.N. (1991) Systemic alpha-adrenergic blockade with phentolamine: a diagnostic test for sympathetically maintained pain. *Anesthesiology*, **74** (4), 691–698.

16 Dubuisson, D. (1989) Effect of dorsal-column stimulation on gelatinosa and marginal neurons of cat spinal cord. *Journal of Neurosurgery*, **70** (2), 257–265.

17 Cui, J.G., O'Connor, W.T., Ungerstedt, U. *et al.* (1997) Spinal cord stimulation attenuates augmented dorsal horn release of excitatory amino acids in mononeuropathy via a GABAergic mechanism. *Pain*, **73** (1), 87–95.

18 Melzack, R. & Wall, P.D. (1965) Pain mechanisms: a new theory. *Science*, **150** (3699), 971–979.

19 Kumar, K., Hunter, G. & Demeria, D. (2006) Spinal cord stimulation in treatment of chronic benign pain: challenges in treatment planning and present status, a 22-year experience. *Neurosurgery*, **58** (3), 481–496; discussion -96.

20 Taylor, R.S., Van Buyten, J.P. & Buchser, E. (2006) Spinal cord stimulation for complex regional pain syndrome: a systematic review of the clinical and cost-effectiveness literature and assessment of prognostic factors. *European Journal of Pain*, **10** (2), 91–101.

21 Kemler, M.A., Raphael, J.H., Bentley, A. & Taylor, R.S. (2010) The cost-effectiveness of spinal cord stimulation for complex regional pain syndrome. *Value in Health*, **13** (6), 735–742.

22 Kemler, M.A., de Vet, H.C., Barendse, G.A. *et al.* (2008) Effect of spinal cord stimulation for chronic complex regional pain syndrome Type I: five-year final follow-up of patients in a randomized controlled trial. *Journal of Neurosurgery*, **108** (2), 292–298.

23 Sears, N.C., Machado, A.G., Nagel, S.J. *et al.* (2011) Long-term outcomes of spinal cord stimulation with paddle leads in the treatment of complex regional pain syndrome and failed back surgery syndrome. *Neuromodulation*, **14** (4), 312–318.

24 Harke, H., Gretenkort, P., Ladleif, H.U. & Rahman, S. (2005) Spinal cord stimulation in sympathetically maintained complex regional pain syndrome type I with severe disability. A prospective clinical study. *European Journal of Pain*, **9** (4), 363–373.

25 van Eijs, F., Geurts, J.W., Van Zundert, J. *et al.* (2012) Spinal cord stimulation in complex regional pain syndrome type I of less than 12-month duration. *Neuromodulation*, **15** (2), 144–150.

Chapter 21

Spinal Cord Stimulation in Other Indications

Konstantin V. Slavin[1] and Sam Eljamel[2]

[1]University of Illinois at Chicago, Chicago, Illinois, USA
[2]University of Dundee, Ninewells Hospital and Medical School, Dundee, UK

Introduction

Spinal cord stimulation (SCS) had been tried in many other disabling conditions with variable outcome. The previous chapters highlighted how successful and cost effective SCS is in failed back surgery syndrome and complex regional pain syndrome. This chapter will summarize other uses of SCS. These off-label indications of SCS are listed in Table 21.1.

Motor control

Beneficial effects of SCS on spasticity were discovered in the 1970s, when several reports documented improvements in spasticity by SCS. Objective evaluation of stretch and H reflexes was used to support clinical results [1], and the most responsive cause of spasticity was dysfunction of the spinal cord due to injury or demyelination [2]. Developed as an alternative to destructive interventions [3,4], SCS has been used in many clinical centers throughout Europe, Asia, and America with impressive long-term results [5,6,7,8]. In addition to patients with spinal cord injuries, SCS has been tried in patients with multiple sclerosis, post-stroke hemiparesis, dystonia, and cerebral palsy. Animal experiments were used to confirm clinical observations and to find an explanation for the SCS effect and putative mechanism of SCS action in these circumstances [9].

It has been postulated that spasticity may be relieved with electrical inhibition of impulses transmitted through the reticulospinal tract. The anterior

Neurostimulation: Principles and Practice, First Edition. Edited by Sam Eljamel and Konstantin V. Slavin.
© 2013 John Wiley & Sons, Ltd. Published 2013 by John Wiley & Sons, Ltd.

Table 21.1 Off-label use of spinal cord stimulation

Motors	Vascular	Genitourinary	Other
Spasticity after stroke, spinal cord injury or demyelination	Peripheral vascular disease	Neurogenic bladder and urinary incontinence	Autonomic hyperreflexia
Cerebral palsy	Unstable angina and ischemic heart disease	Female orgasmic dysfunction	Minimally responsive state
Parkinson's disease	Cerebral ischemia		Brain tumors
Cervical dystonia			Radiation-induced brain injury

location of the reticulospinal tract in the spinal cord does not allow direct stimulation of this structure from the posterior epidural space without impulses traveling through the dorsal columns. This may explain the following observations:

(1) The observed need in higher than usual settings for spasticity control.
(2) The fact that paresthesia coverage may not correlate with spasticity relief.
(3) The spasticity control seems to be more pronounced in patients with more advanced stages of demyelination when sensory impairment allows higher electrical stimulation parameters to be utilized.

Although the initial impression suggested that spasticity of cerebral origin does not respond to SCS [2], subsequent studies showed sustained benefits of SCS in patients with post-stroke weakness [10,11], dystonia [12], and post-hypoxic encephalopathy [13]. The general enthusiasm was lowered by reports indicating a lack of clinical long-term effectiveness [14,15] or cost-effectiveness of SCS in spasticity [16], but the main reason for almost complete abandonment of SCS in spasticity was the introduction of intrathecal baclofen administration [17]. However, in those countries where intrathecal baclofen is not available because of regulatory barriers, SCS remains a useful tool for treatment of otherwise refractory spasticity through non-destructive intervention [18,19].

In addition to suppression of spasticity in symptomatic patients, SCS may be effective in the recovery of motor function in paraplegic patients. A study of 10 patients with complete motor spinal cord injury indicated that epidural SCS at the lumbosacral spinal cord level recruited leg muscles in a segmental-selective way generating integrated motor behavior of sustained extension and rhythmic flexion and extension movements [20]. In a case of incomplete spinal cord injury, a wheelchair-dependent patient was able to walk with a walker essentially in an effortless manner after prolonged SCS. The superiority of gait assisted by SCS was particularly impressive in ambulation at longer distances [21].

The latest surge of interest in SCS for treatment of motor disorders has come from experimental study showing improvement in locomotion in an experimental model of Parkinson disease (PD) [22]. The improvement in mobility and restoration of normal patterns of neuronal activity were observed with dorsal column stimulation in both the acute PD model of pharmacologically dopamine-depleted mice and chronic PD model of hydroxydopamine lesioned rats [22].

Vasoactive applications of spinal cord stimulation

With the primary intent of pain relief, early SCS implanters noticed that in addition to paresthesias and/or sense of vibration, patients described a sensation of warmth in their extremities, and along with this subjective sensation there may have been objective vasodilatation and blood flow augmentation. As early as 1976, several groups had described changes in peripheral blood flow in response to SCS, laying the foundation for subsequent widespread clinical applications [23,24].

This consistent and reproducible effect on autonomic functions became the basis of SCS application for blood flow augmentation and ischemic pain relief in the treatment of vascular disorders such as peripheral arterial occlusive disease [25], coronary ischemia/intractable angina (IA) [26], and vasospastic disease in the extremities [27].

The use of SCS to treat peripheral vascular disease (PVD) was started in 1976, when substantial relief of vascular pain was reported in nine patients [23]. Eleven years later, Murphy and Giles [28] published similar results in 10 patients suffering from IA. Within a few years, SCS was widely used all over the world. However, the initial good results reported in carefully selected patients suffering from PVD and IA, along with the non-destructive and fully reversible nature of SCS treatment, led to indiscriminate clinical applications and, accordingly, to poorer clinical results. A systematic review [29,30] of controlled studies comparing SCS with any form of conservative treatment in patients with inoperable PVD found significantly higher limb salvage rates after 12 months, more pronounced pain relief, and a significantly better chance of reaching Fontaine stage II in SCS-treated patients. Moreover, persistent benefits beyond the first year of treatment, as shown by a limb salvage rate of 78% after 5 years of SCS treatment in 24 long-term survivors, has been reported [31].

The efficacy of SCS in IA is mostly supported by various randomized trials, one placebo-controlled study, and several controlled trials [32]. Out of 104 patients with triple vessel coronary disease randomly assigned to either SCS treatment or to coronary artery bypass grafting (CABG), Mannheimer et al. [33] found at 6 months postoperatively less mortality ($p = 0.02$) in SCS patients, and equivalent symptom relief in both groups, albeit better exercise capacity ($p = 0.02$) after CABG. Follow-up investigation of the same patients at 5 years found identical mortality in both groups [34]. In contrast, longitudinal studies have failed to demonstrate any influence of SCS treatment on left ventricular function [35] or cardiac arrhythmias [36]. Finally, the fear that SCS could deprive the patient of a vital warning signal and thus favor the development of cardiac ischemia and myocardial infarction has vanished over time because all available literature has established that SCS raises anginal threshold without eliminating the typical pain from IA or symptoms of myocardial infarction. Furthermore, long-term studies including a large number of patients have concluded that SCS neither adversely affects mortality nor morbidity [37,38,39].

Genitourinary effects of spinal cord stimulation

Conus medullaris SCS for micturition control in a paraplegic patient was first performed in 1970; this approach was later used in a group of another 10 paraplegic patients with long-lasting symptomatic improvement [40]. Improved bladder control was one of the major results of SCS in a group of 24 patients with upper motor neuron disease, including multiple sclerosis, traumatic spinal cord injury, and neurodegenerative conditions [41], and another group of 11 patients with multiple sclerosis [42].

When SCS was implanted specifically to treat neurogenic bladder, most patients developed complete or almost complete normalization of urination with relief of bladder spasticity, marked increase in bladder capacity, and reduction or abolition of post-void residual urine volume [43]. The same group of authors noticed no changes in bladder striatal activity or detrusor reflexes in those patients who underwent SCS for pain treatment and had intact bladder function [43].

The urodynamic changes do not occur in all patients undergoing SCS: in a study of patients with spinal cord injury who underwent SCS implantation for control of spasticity, less than 20% (6 out of 33) were found to have changes in lower urinary tract function [44].

In addition to bladder function normalization, SCS appears to facilitate normalization of bowel regimen and morning erections in a group of patients with post-traumatic paraplegia [3].

In a somewhat unconventional approach, SCS was used to treat female orgasmic dysfunction [45]. In this series of 11 patients, a single percutaneous SCS electrode was used to produce pleasurable genital stimulation and subsequent orgasm. In 91% of subjects, SCS resulted in increased lubrication, greater frequency in sexual activity, and overall satisfaction. An orgasmic capacity returned in 80% of patients with secondary anorgasmia while using SCS, but anorgasmia returned once the device was removed. Despite pleasurable paresthesias in the genital area, none of the patients with primary anorgasmia (those who never had an orgasm) experienced orgasm during the study, making the researchers speculate on whether the underlying difficulty that prevented orgasm from occurring throughout the patient's life could not be overcome with SCS application. At the same time, the possibility of a longer stimulation period (longer than 9 days) resolving primary anorgasmia was also brought up [44].

Other areas of spinal cord stimulation application

Impaired consciousness

Anecdotal reports of SCS in the treatment of impaired consciousness exist. Out of eight patients with severe brain dysfunction due to head injury, vasospasm, or tumor resection, two regained consciousness and speech after 1-2 months of high cervical SCS [45]. The patients were implanted with a four-contact paddle electrode at the C2-4 level and stimulation was delivered twice a day for 4 h. The authors concluded that SCS may accelerate the natural course of recovery in patients after brain injury.

In the treatment of vegetative state, eight out of 23 patients who underwent SCS exhibited symptomatic improvement, and seven of these were able to follow verbal orders [46]. It was noted that onset of improvement varied from the first few weeks to as long as 10-12 months after SCS initiation. There was significant improvement in cerebral blood flow associated with SCS in some of the patients, but this phenomenon did not correlate with clinical improvement.

The mechanism of symptomatic improvement is largely unclear, but positron emission tomography (PET) revealed changes in glucose consumption in two patients with prolonged post-traumatic unconsciousness [47]. A patient who improved clinically had higher glucose uptake in the brainstem, hypothalamic, thalamic, and certain cortical regions, while the other patient whose consciousness did not improve had no or minimal changes in glucose uptake.

SCS was investigated as an early stage intervention in patients with hypoxic encephalopathy [48]. The SCS electrode was inserted and therapy was started within a month after the hypoxic event in 12 patients ranging in age from 7 to 72 years. An improvement was observed in 58% of patients within 2 weeks after starting SCS. Although there was an improvement in the ability to communicate with others and to express emotions, disturbances of writing, picture drawing, and calculation were not improved by SCS stimulation.

In a recent update, based on clinical experience of more than 200 patients treated with SCS for impaired consciousness, SCS may work in young patients with a history of brain trauma and evidence of brain atrophy with no other major lesions and cerebral flow (CBF) values of 20 mL/100 g/min or higher [49]. Out of 15 patients who satisfied all the above criteria for SCS, 12 improved with SCS, and seven of these improved significantly, thereby indicating that SCS was effective in 80% of this selected patient group [49].

Another direction recently explored involved combination of high cervical SCS and hyperbaric oxygenation (HBO) in 12 patients whose coma lasted more than 3 months [50]. Six patients (50%) emerged from coma as a result of combined treatment and regained consciousness. SCS was delivered through four-contact paddle electrodes and the stimulation regimen was set as 15 min on/15 min off for a duration of 14 h during the daytime. It is, however, unclear whether SCS or HBO was responsible for symptomatic improvement, as every patient who emerged from the vegetative state did so within the first 6 months of treatment during or soon after the period when both SCS and HBO were administered, and there were no additional dramatic improvements when SCS was used alone [51].

Autonomic hyperreflexia

Autonomic hyperreflexia, a frequent and difficult to manage symptom of spinal cord injury, was significantly reduced or eliminated in four out of five patients implanted with SCS [52].

Spinal cord stimulation and cerebral blood flow

Although the mechanism of vasoregulation appears different between cerebral and peripheral or coronary circulations, the ability of SCS to augment peripheral and coronary blood flow was tested in regard to CBF in the mid-1980s. Similar to other fields of SCS use, human experience preceded animal studies. In 1985, Hosobuchi [53] found that SCS at upper cervical levels could increase CBF. The same result was not found with stimulation of thoracic levels. Later, the same author tested cervical SCS in three patients with symptomatic cerebral ischemia (one with anterior and two with posterior circulation occlusion), and although good results were obtained, further studies are needed to confirm its clinical application [54].

Several animal experiments in rats, cats, rabbits, and dogs [55–63] have shown augmentation of CBF with cervical SCS. The level of stimulation seemed to have a direct effect on the blood flow, with stimulation of upper levels (C1–3) generating higher flow values.

Using a cat model, a group from Japan showed that CBF augmentation with cervical SCS is no longer observed after sectioning of the dorsal columns at the cervicomedullary junction [55]. The authors postulated that CBF is increased from cervical SCS mainly through a central pathway. Similar results were obtained by another group of researchers using rat model [59]. The researchers demonstrated lack of changes in CBF after resection of the superior cervical ganglion while using SCS.

Researchers from Italy demonstrated that SCS could increase, decrease, or have no effect in CBF [64]. The difference correlated mainly with the stimulated level of the spinal cord. Thoracic stimulation had a low effect and sometimes even decreased CBF. Cervical stimulation more frequently produced CBF augmentation (61%). In another study, the same group found that vasoconstriction of the carotid arteries with sympathetic trunk stimulation was attenuated by cervical SCS [65]. In this experiment they used a rabbit model to observe CBF changes with SCS alone, sympathetic trunk stimulation alone, and simultaneous spinal cord and sympathetic trunk stimulation.

The hypothetic treatment for cerebral vasospasm after subarachnoid hemorrhage (SAH) with SCS has been tried in different animal models. Increased blood flow was found in rats with SAH and SCS compared with control groups [57]. Similarly, prevention of early vasospasm was described in rabbits treated with SCS after induced SAH [66]. Recently, the vasodilatation effect of SCS was shown in the basilar artery of rats 5 days after induction of SAH. Radiotracer studies, laser Doppler flowmetry, and histologic photomicrographs were used to prove these changes in the delayed spasm [62].

Based on experimental data, several possible mechanisms for SCS action in prevention and treatment of SAH-related vasospasm were hypothesized; it is conceivable that stimulation at different levels of the cervical spinal cord will result in different clinical effects [67]. In theory, stimulation of the lower cervical spinal cord may allow vasospasm to be prevented by acting through modulation of sympathetic activity, essentially constituting a functional, temporary sympathectomy, and preventing cerebral arteries from vasoconstriction after SAH. But once the vasospasm is present, the patient may receive additional benefit and possibly improve clinical outcome by CBF augmentation and treatment of the vasospasm by stimulation of the upper cervical spinal cord, possibly acting through more central, medullary mechanisms that are responsible for immediate vasospasm after SAH and for subsequent vasodilatation needed for vasospasm treatment [67].

A pioneering study related to the use of SCS for cerebral vasospasm in humans was performed in the late 1990s in Japan [68]. Ten SAH patients with secured cerebral aneurysm were implanted with percutaneous quadripolar epidural cervical leads. The stimulation was continuous and started on day 5 (±1) post bleeding for 10-15 days. CBF was measured with xenon computed tomography; it was significantly increased in the distribution of the middle cerebral artery with SCS. Four patients presented with angiographic vasospasm and three were reported with clinical vasospasm. One patient died and the overall outcome was good or excellent in seven. No major adverse effect was attributed to the use of SCS. The data analysis correlated the increase in CBF with SCS.

To prove the concept, Slavin et al. [51] recently performed a prospective safety/feasibility study of cervical SCS in prevention/treatment of cerebral vasospasm after aneurysmal SAH. In the study, 12 patients were implanted with percutaneous eight-contact SCS electrodes immediately upon completion of the aneurysm-securing procedure, either clipping or coiling, while the patient was still under general anesthesia. By the study protocol, SCS had to be initiated the following morning and within 72 h after SAH, and then administered continuously for 14 consecutive days. The authors found that cervical SCS was safe and feasible as there were no complications related to the electrode insertion or the stimulation itself. One patient died during the study from unrelated causes, and two electrodes were pulled out prematurely. Angiographic vasospasm was observed in six out of 12 patients, and clinical vasospasm in two out of 12. Both incidences were smaller than predicted based on Fisher, and Hunt and Hess grades, although this incidence reduction did not reach statistical significance. There were no long-term side effects of SCS during 1 year of follow-up. Subsequent data analysis indicated that preventive effects of cervical SCS on vasospasm might correlate with the stimulated level [69].

In addition to acute ischemia from cerebral vasospasm, SCS has been shown to increase CBF in chronic ischemic conditions. The results were encouraging in the patients with chronic vascular occlusion [54], and in a case of old cerebral infarction, SCS resulted in a dramatic increase of blood flow velocities measured by transcranial Doppler [70].

Spinal cord stimulation and brain tumors

In a novel application of SCS, SCS at the cervical level was shown to increase local blood flow in patients with brain tumors [71]. This phenomenon was then used in a clinical series of 23 patients with high-grade malignant brain tumors [72]. Based on the known association between hypoxia and low perfusion in malignant neoplasms and resistance to radiotherapy, and significant increase in tumor radiosensitivity with increased local tissue oxygenation, the researchers postulated that SCS with its augmentation of CBF and ability to increase glucose metabolism might improve treatment outcome in high-grade gliomas. The preliminary results of this application of SCS were described as promising, and blood flow and glucose metabolism have been consistently higher in patients with high-grade gliomas undergoing continuous high cervical SCS [72]. In this patient group, a single four-contact percutaneous SCS electrode was placed over the dorsal surface of the spinal cord at the C2–4 level, and stimulation was delivered at an amplitude of 3 V or less, producing mild paresthesias in upper extremities.

Spinal cord stimulation and radiation-induced brain injury

Since hypoxia and impaired tissue perfusion are hallmarks for radiation-induced brain injury, high cervical SCS was used to improve glucose metabolism in a prospective series of eight patients [73]. As glucose metabolism increased by about 40% as a result of SCS stimulation, the authors noted a reduction in corticosteroid requirements in patients without concurrent tumor. These results may offer a new avenue for treatment of radiation-induced brain injury, perhaps decreasing or eliminating the need for radical surgical interventions for this frustrating and hard-to-manage complication.

Conclusions

Although SCS is primarily used for the control of chronic pain, interest in SCS applications for a variety of other indications continues to grow. In the constantly changing field of neuromodulation, some indications disappear due to advancement of competing approaches (as in the case of intrathecal baclofen replacing SCS use for treatment of spasticity), while others become more promising. The use of SCS for treatment of PD, for example, may be a less invasive alternative to DBS.

The use of SCS for peripheral vascular disease and intractable angina remains extremely common in Europe, but the lack of FDA approval has prevented its widespread acceptance in the USA.

SCS for minimally conscious and vegetative state may be used before considering more invasive approaches such as deep brain stimulation.

In the field of genitourinary conditions, sacral nerve stimulation may be augmented in some patients with SCS, and changes in sexual function may become another common use of this technology if the anecdotal published experience is confirmed by larger clinical series.

The newer and promising indications such as cerebral vasospasm have a potential of significant improvement in morbidity and mortality in a very difficult patient category, while other directions such as SCS for brain tumors are still in their infancy with a rather uncertain future.

References

1 Siegfried, J., Krainick, J.U., Haas, H. *et al.* (1978) Electrical spinal cord stimulation for spastic movement disorders. *Applied Neurophysiology*, **41**, 134-141.

2 Siegfried, J. (1980) Treatment of spasticity by dorsal cord stimulation. *International Rehabilitation Medicine*, **2**, 31-34.

3 Richardson, R.R., Cerullo, L.J., McLone, D.G. *et al.* (1979) Percutaneous epidural neurostimulation in modulation of paraplegic spasticity. Six case reports. *Acta Neurochirurgica*, **49**, 235-243.

4 Barolat, G. (1988) Surgical management of spasticity and spasms in spinal cord injury: an overview. *The Journal of the American Paraplegia Society*, **11**, 9-13.

5 Reynolds, A.F. & Oakley, J.C. (1982) High frequency cervical epidural stimulation for spasticity. *Applied Neurophysiology*, **45**, 93-97.

6 Koulousakis, A., Buchhaas, U. & Nittner, K. (1987) Application of SCS for movement disorders and spasticity. *Acta Neurochirurgica. Supplementum*, **39**, 112-116.

7 Barolat, G., Myklebust, J.B. & Wenninger, W. (1988) Effects of spinal cord stimulation on spasticity and spasms secondary to myelopathy. *Applied Neurophysiology*, **51** (1), 29-44.

8 Kanaka, T.S. & Kumar, M.M. (1990) Neural stimulation for spinal spasticity. *Paraplegia*, **28**, 399-405.

9 Maiman, D.J., Mykleburst, J.B. & Barolat-Romana, G. (1987) Spinal cord stimulation for amelioration of spasticity: experimental results. *Neurosurgery*, **21**, 331-333.

10 Nakamura, S. & Tsubokawa, T. (1985) Evaluation of spinal cord stimulation for postapoplectic spastic hemiplegia. *Neurosurgery*, **17**, 253-259.

11 Cioni, B. & Meglio, M. (1987) Spinal cord stimulation improves motor performances in hemiplegics: clinical and neurophysiological study. *Acta Neurochirurgica. Supplementum*, **39**, 103-105.

12 Goetz, C.G., Penn, R.D. & Tanner, C.M. (1988) Efficacy of cervical cord stimulation in dystonia. *Advances in Neurology*, **50**, 645-649.

13 Terao, T., Taya, K., Sawauchi, S. *et al.* (2004) Therapeutic effect of spinal cord stimulation for a patient suffering spasticity after hypoxia of the brain. *No Shinkei Geka. Neurological Surgery*, **32**, 613-618.

14 Gottlieb, G.L., Myklebust, B.M., Stefoski, D. *et al.* (1985) Evaluation of cervical stimulation for chronic treatment of spasticity. *Neurology*, **35**, 699-704.

15 Hugenholtz, H., Humphreys, P., McIntyre, W.M. *et al.* (1988) Cervical spinal cord stimulation for spasticity in cerebral palsy. *Neurosurgery*, **22**, 707-714.

16 Midha, M. & Schmitt, J.K. (1998) Epidural spinal cord stimulation for the control of spasticity in spinal cord injury patients lacks long-term efficacy and is not cost-effective. *Spinal Cord*, **36**, 190-192.

17 Lazorthes, Y., Sol, J.C., Sallerin, B. *et al.* (2002) The surgical management of spasticity. *European Journal of Neurology*, **9** (Suppl. 1), 35-41; discussion 53-61.

18 Shabalov, V.A., Bril', A.G., Kurenkov, A.L. *et al.* (2000) The use of chronic epidural electrostimulation of the spinal cord in children with spastic diplegia-a type of infantile cerebral palsy. *Zhurnal Voprosy Neirokhirurgii Imeni N. N. Burdenko*, **3**, 2-6.

19 Shabalov, V.A., Dekopov, A.V. & Troshina, E.M. (2006) Preliminary results of treatment for spastic forms of infantile cerebral paralysis by chronic epidural neurostimulation of lumbar enlargement. *Zhurnal Voprosy Neirokhirurgii Imeni N. N. Burdenko*, **3**, 10-13.

20 Minassian, K., Jilge, B., Rattay, F. *et al.* (2004) Stepping like movements in humans with complete spinal cord injury induced by epidural stimulation of the lumbar cord: electromyographic study of compound muscle action potentials. *Spinal Cord*, **42**, 401-416.

21 Herman, R., He, J., D'Luzansky, S. *et al.* (2002) Spinal cord stimulation facilitates functional walking in a chronic, incomplete spinal cord injured. *Spinal Cord*, **40**, 65-68.

22 Fuentes, R., Petersson, P., Siesser, W.B. *et al.* (2009) Spinal cord stimulation restores locomotion in animal models of Parkinson's disease. *Science*, **323**, 1578-1582.

23 Dooley, D.M. & Kasprak, M. (1976) Modification of blood flow to the extremities by electrical stimulation of the nervous system. *Southern Medical Journal*, **69**, 1309-1311.

24 Cook, A.W., Oygar, A., Baggenstos, P. *et al.* (1976) Vascular disease of extremities. Electric stimulation of spinal cord and posterior roots. *New York State Journal of Medicine*, **76**, 366-368.

25 Vincenzo, S. & Kyventidis, T. (2007) Epidural spinal cord stimulation in lower limb ischemia. *Acta Neurochirurgica. Supplement*, **97** (1), 253-258.

26 Hautvast, R.W., Blanksma, P.K., DeJongste, M.J. *et al.* (1996) Effect of spinal cord stimulation on myocardial blood flow assessed by positron emission tomography in patients with refractory angina pectoris. *The American Journal of Cardiology*, **77**, 462-467.

27 Robaina, F.J., Dominguez, M., Diaz, M. *et al.* (1989) Spinal cord stimulation for relief of chronic pain in vasospastic disorders of the upper limbs. *Neurosurgery*, **24**, 63-67.

28 Murphy, D. & Giles, K. (1987) Dorsal column stimulation for pain relief from intractable angina pectoris. *Pain*, **28**, 365-368.

29 Ubbink, D.T. & Vermeulen, H. (2003) Spinal cord stimulation for non-reconstructable chronic critical limb ischemia. *Cochrane Database Systematic Review* **3**:CD004001.

30 Amann, W., Berg, P., Gersbach, P. *et al.*, for the SCS-EPOS Study Group (2003) Spinal cord stimulation in the treatment of non-reconstructable stable critical leg ischemia: results of the European peripheral vascular disease outcome study (SCS-EPOS). *European Journal of Vascular and Endovascular Surgery*, **26**, 280–286.

31 Gersbach, P.A., Argitis, V., Gardaz, J.-P., von Segesser, L.K. & Haesler, E. (2007) Late outcome of spinal cord stimulation for unreconstructable and limbthreatening lower limb ischemia. *European Journal of Vascular and Endovascular Surgery*, **33**, 717–724.

32 Nashold, B.S., Jr, Grimes, J., Friedman, H., Semans, J. & Avery, R. (1977-8) Electrical stimulation of the conus medullaris in the paraplegic. A 5-year review. *Applied Neurophysiology*, **40**, 192–207.

33 Mannheimer, C., Eliasson, T., Augustinsson, L.E. *et al.* (1998) Electrical stimulation versus coronary artery bypass surgery in severe angina pectoris. The ESBY study. *Circulation*, **97**, 1157–1163.

34 Ekre, O., Eliasson, T., Norsell, H. *et al.* (2002) Long-term effects of spinal cord stimulation and coronary artery bypass grafting on quality of life and survival in the ESBY study. *European Heart Journal*, **23**, 1938–1945.

35 Hautvast, R.W., Szabo, B.M., DeJongste, M.J.L. *et al.* (1993) Influence of spinal cord stimulation on left ventricular function in patients with refractory angina pectoris, 2nd International Symposium on Heart Failure-mechanisms and management.

36 Eliasson, T., Augustinsson, L.E. & Mannheimer, C. (1996) Spinal cord stimulation in severe angina pectoris – presentation of current studies, indications, and clinical experience. *Pain*, **65**, 169–179.

37 Greco, S., Auriti, A., Fiume, D. *et al.* (1999) Spinal cord stimulation for the treatment of refractory angina pectoris: a two-year follow-up. *Pacing and Clinical Electrophysiology*, **22**, 26–32.

38 Ten Vaarwerk, I., Jessurun, G., de Jongste, M. *et al.* (1999) Clinical outcome of patients treated with spinal cord stimulation for therapeutically refractory angina pectoris. *Heart (British Cardiac Society)*, **82**, 82–88.

39 Jacobs, M.J.H.M., Jörning, P.J.G., Beckers, R.C.Y. *et al.* (1990) Foot salvage and improvement of microvascular blood flow as a result of epidural spinal cord electrical stimulation. *Journal of Vascular Surgery*, **12**, 354–360.

40 Campos, R.J., Dimitrijevic, M.M., Faganel, J. *et al.* (1981) Clinical evaluation of the effect of spinal cord stimulation on motor performance in patients with upper motor neuron lesions. *Applied Neurophysiology*, **44**, 141–151.

41 Read, D.J., Matthews, W.B. & Higson, R.H. (1980) The effect of spinal cord stimulation on function in patients with multiple sclerosis. *Brain: A Journal of Neurology*, **103**, 803–833.

42 Meglio, M., Cioni, B., Amico, E.D. *et al.* (1980) Epidural spinal cord stimulation for the treatment of neurogenic bladder. *Acta Neurochirurgica*, **54**, 191–199.

43 Katz, P.G., Greenstein, A., Severs, S.L. *et al.* (1991) Effect of implanted epidural stimulator on lower urinary tract function in spinal-cord-injured patients. *European Urology*, **20**, 103–106.

44 Meloy, T.S. & Southern, J.P. (2006) Neurally augmented sexual function in human females: a preliminary investigation. *Neuromodulation*, **9**, 34–40.

45 Matsui, T., Asano, T., Takakura, K. *et al.* (1989) Beneficial effects of cervical spinal cord stimulation (cSCS) on patients with impaired consciousness: a preliminary report. *Pacing and Clinical Electrophysiology*, **12**, 718–725.

46 Kanno, T., Kamel, U., Yokoyama, T. *et al.* (1989) Effects of dorsal column spinal cord stimulation on reversibility of neuronal function. Experience of

treatment for vegetative states. *Pacing and Clinical Electrophysiology*, **12**, 733-738.

47 Yamaguchi, N., Seki, H., Ikeda, K. *et al.* (1995) Effects of cervical spinal cord stimulation in glucose consumption in patients with post traumatic prolonged unconsciousness. *Neurologia Medico-Chirurgica*, **35**, 797-803.

48 Fujii, M., Sadamitsu, D., Maekawa, T. *et al.* (1998) Spinal cord stimulation in an early stage for unresponsive patients with hypoxic encephalopathy. *No Shinkei Geka. Neurological Surgery*, **26**, 315-321.

49 Morita, I., Keith, M.W. & Kanno, T. (2007) Dorsal column stimulation for persistent vegetative state. *Acta Neurochirurgica. Supplement*, **97** (1), 455-459.

50 Liu, J.T., Lee, J.K., Tyan, Y.S. *et al.* (2009) Neuromodulation on cervical spinal cord combined with hyperbaric oxygen in comatose patients—a preliminary report. *Surgical Neurology*, **72** (S2), 28-34.

51 Slavin, K.V. (2009) Commentary to Liu *et al.* (39). *Surgical Neurology*, **72** (S2), 34-35.

52 Richardson, R.R., Cerullo, L.J. & Meyer, P.R. (1979) Autonomic hyper-reflexia modulated by percutaneous epidural neurostimulation: a preliminary report. *Neurosurgery*, **4**, 517-520.

53 Hosobuchi, Y. (1985) Electrical stimulation of the cervical spinal cord increases cerebral blood flow in humans. *Applied Neurophysiology*, **48**, 372-376.

54 Hosobuchi, Y. (1991) Treatment of cerebral ischemia with electrical stimulation of the cervical spinal cord. *Pacing and Clinical Electrophysiology*, **14**, 122-126.

55 Isono, M., Kaga, A., Fujiki, M. *et al.* (1995) Effect of spinal cord stimulation on cerebral blood flow in cats. *Stereotactic and Functional Neurosurgery*, **64**, 40-46.

56 Sagher, O. & Huang, D.L. (2000) Effects of cervical spinal cord stimulation on cerebral blood flow in the rat. *Journal of Neurosurgery*, **93** (Suppl. 1), 71-76.

57 Ebel, H., Schomäcker, K., Balogh, A. *et al.* (2001) High cervical spinal cord stimulation (CSCS) increases regional cerebral blood flow after induced subarachnoid haemorrhage in rats. *Minimally Invasive Neurosurgery*, **44**, 167-171.

58 Patel, S., Huang, D.L. & Sagher, O. (2003) Sympathetic mechanisms in cerebral blood flow alterations induced by spinal cord stimulation. *Journal of Neurosurgery*, **99**, 754-761.

59 Patel, S., Huang, D.L. & Sagher, O. (2004) Evidence for a central pathway in the cerebrovascular effects of spinal cord stimulation. *Neurosurgery*, **55**, 201-206.

60 Gurelik, M., Kayabas, M., Karadag, O. *et al.* (2005) Cervical spinal cord stimulation improves neurological dysfunction induced by cerebral vasospasm. *Neuroscience*, **134**, 827-832.

61 Karadağ, Ö., Eroğlu, E., Gürelik, M. *et al.* (2005) Cervical spinal cord stimulation increases cerebral cortical blood flow in an experimental vasospasm model. *Acta Neurochirurgica*, **147**, 79-84.

62 Lee, J.Y., Huang, D.L., Keep, R. *et al.* (2008) Effect of electrical stimulation of the cervical spinal cord on blood flow following subarachnoid hemorrhage. *Journal of Neurosurgery*, **109**, 1148-1154.

63 Yang, X., Farber, J.P., Wu, M. *et al.* (2008) Roles of dorsal column pathway and transient receptor potential vanilloid type 1 in augmentation of cerebral blood flow by upper cervical spinal cord stimulation in rats. *Neuroscience*, **152**, 950-958.

64 Visocchi, M. (2006) Spinal cord stimulation and cerebral haemodynamics. *Acta Neurochirurgica. Supplement*, **99**, 111-116.

65 Visocchi, M., Cioni, B., Vergari, S. *et al.* (1994) Spinal cord stimulation and cerebral blood flow: an experimental study. *Stereotactic and Functional Neurosurgery*, **62**, 186-190.

66 Visocchi, M., Argiolas, L., Meglio, M. *et al.* (2001) Spinal cord stimulation and early experimental cerebral spasm: the "functional monitoring" and the "preventing effect". *Acta Neurochirurgica*, **143**, 177-185.

67 Goellner, E. & Slavin, K.V. (2009) Cervical spinal cord stimulation may prevent cerebral vasospasm by modulating sympathetic activity of the superior cervical ganglion at lower cervical spinal level. *Medical Hypotheses*, **73**, 410-413.

68 Takanashi, Y. & Shinonaga, M. (2000) Spinal cord stimulation for cerebral vasospasm as prophylaxis. *Neurologia Medico-Chirurgica*, **40**, 352-356.

69 Slavin, K.V., Goellner, E., Eboli, P. *et al.* (2009) Cervical spinal cord stimulation for prevention of cerebral vasospasm in aneurysmal subarachnoid haemorrhage: preliminary results of first North American study. *Journal of Cerebral Blood Flow & Metabolism*, **29**, S308.

70 Visocchi, M., Cioni, B., Pentimalli, L. *et al.* (1994) Increase of cerebral blood flow and improvement of brain motor control following spinal cord stimulation in ischemic spastic hemiparesis. *Stereotactic and Functional Neurosurgery*, **62**, 103-107.

71 Clavo, B., Robaina, F., Catalá, L. *et al.* (2003) Increased locoregional blood flow in brain tumors after cervical spinal cord stimulation. *Journal of Neurosurgery*, **98**, 1263-1270.

72 Robaina, F. & Clavo, B. (2007) The role of spinal cord stimulation in the management of patients with brain tumors. *Acta Neurochirurgica. Supplement*, **97** (1), 445-453.

73 Clavo, B., Robaina, F., Montz, R. *et al.* (2009) Modification of glucose metabolism in radiation-induced brain injury areas using cervical spinal cord stimulation. *Acta Neurochirurgica*, **151**, 1419-1425.

Part 5
Peripheral Nerve Stimulation

Chapter 22

Peripheral Nerve Stimulation in Head and Face Pain

Konstantin V. Slavin[1], Serge Y. Rasskazoff[2], and Sami Al-Nafi[1]

[1]University of Illinois at Chicago, Chicago, Illinois, USA
[2]Flint, Michigan, USA

Introduction

The term peripheral nerve stimulation (PNS) refers to electrical neuromodulation that involves delivery of repetitive low-power electrical impulses directly to the fibers of a peripheral nerve. The difference between PNS and transcutaneous electrical nerve stimulation (TENS) and percutaneous electrical nerve stimulation (PENS) is that PNS involves long-term use of implanted devices (electrode leads) that are placed in the vicinity of a peripheral nerve or in direct contact with the nerve trunk, whereas TENS delivers electrical impulses through the skin and PENS uses electrodes that are inserted only for the period of stimulation session. There are several other terms that are associated with specific technical or anatomical nuances but sometimes used interchangeably with PNS or are considered a variation of PNS. These include subcutaneous peripheral nerve stimulation, peripheral nerve field stimulation, or simply peripheral field stimulation, and usually they refer to stimulation of peripheral field of pain rather than a certain named nerve, although the principle of the approach is similar. Interested readers may get more in-depth analysis of different procedural terms by reviewing the articles listed in the Further reading section at the end of this chapter.

PNS in this context refers to the use of this modality to control chronic pain. Other applications of PNS, such as treatment of sphincter dysfunction with pelvic nerve stimulation, diaphragmal palsy with phrenic nerve stimulation, seizures and depression with vagal nerve stimulation, obstructive sleep apnea with hypoglossal nerve stimulation, etc., are either covered by dedicated chapters or are beyond the scope of this book.

Neurostimulation: Principles and Practice, First Edition. Edited by Sam Eljamel and Konstantin V. Slavin.

Historical perspectives and rationale of peripheral nerve stimulation

Although still considered "new and experimental" by some implanters and insurers, PNS is probably neither: it predates the more ubiquitous spinal cord stimulation (SCS). In fact, PNS was used as an illustration of the "gate control" theory of pain back in 1965 when Wall and Sweet [1] stimulated their own infraorbital nerves to demonstrate suppression of pain sensation during electrical stimulation of the nerve trunk. Over the first 25 years of its clinical use, PNS was almost exclusively associated with open surgical interventions when the surgeon exposed a peripheral nerve and implanted a paddle electrode directly over the nerve or next to it [2]. During this period, most surgical indications for PNS, patient selection criteria, and clinical expectations were established. By virtue of this requirement for surgical exploration of the nerve, PNS was used exclusively by surgical specialists, mainly neurosurgeons, but also orthopedic and plastic surgeons with expertise in peripheral nerve surgery. This approach changed in the early 1990s when the percutaneous techniques of PNS electrode insertion in the vicinity of the stimulated nerve were introduced by Weiner and Reed [3]. This invention revolutionized the PNS field: it not only opened the modality to neuromodulation practitioners with a non-surgical background, but also widened the field for many new indications, such as chronic migraines, cluster headaches, axial pain in the neck and back, etc.

The interest in PNS has been growing exponentially over the last two decades, and, by some estimates, the number of PNS trials and implants may be reaching those of SCS in some geographical areas. This is partly due to PNS simplicity and its minimally invasive approach, and partly because of the large number of patients and clinical situations where SCS is not particularly effective (i.e., pain in head and face, axial pain syndromes, abdominal and chest wall pains).

Today, PNS is an established modality in the spectrum of neuromodulation for pain: it is an important part of the neuromodulation continuum that starts from peripheral nerve endings and ends in somatosensory, motor, and limbic cortical areas. Owing to very distinct nuances of PNS in head and face and in the rest of the body, we decided to split this topic into two separate subchapters, each with its own set of indications, technical pearls, complications, and troubleshooting approaches.

Indications for peripheral nerve stimulation in the head and face

Occipital neuralgia

The most established indication for craniofacial PNS is occipital neuralgia (ON), a chronic pain syndrome characterized by stabbing sharp pains in the distribution of the occipital nerve(s). Although there are multiple medical and surgical approaches to treat ON, none of them is uniformly successful. Therefore, the potential treatment of ON with PNS was suggested in the mid-1970s [4]. Since the introduction of the percutaneous approach, PNS has been widely used for ON, and a variety of electrode configurations, combinations and directions has been tried with different degrees of success [3,5]. Even now the neuropathic pain of ON appears to be the most established indication for PNS in the craniofacial region.

Trigeminal neuropathic pain

Trigeminal neuropathic pain (TNP) represents a chronic pain syndrome that combines sharp or dull pain in the distribution of one or several branches of the trigeminal nerve and usually involves a combination of constant and episodic pain. TNP is associated with some degree of sensory impairment and usually follows a traumatic or surgical event such as sinus surgery and facial injury. There are no reliable surgical interventions for TNP. Various ablative or decompressive procedures, such as neurolysis, neurotomy, neurectomy, and nerve avulsion have been suggested, but most of them offer either temporary improvement, rarely effective, or carry a risk of worsening of both pain and sensory loss. Trigeminal PNS has been used for treatment of TNP in many clinical centers, and there is little controversy that it presents an attractive alternative to neurodestruction in TNP [6,7]. In addition to PNS, neuromodulation of the trigeminal ganglion has been described as a feasible, safe, and effective modality for TNP [8].

Chronic headaches

Severe chronic migraine headaches and trigeminal autonomic cephalgias (cluster headaches, sudden unilateral neuralgiform headache attacks with conjunctival injection and tearing, paroxysmal hemicrania and hemicrania continua) are known for relative unresponsiveness to medical and surgical treatments in a number of patients. These patients are considered treatment refractory. Although treatment-refractory migraine patients represent only a small percentage of all migraine sufferers, this represent hundreds in real terms because of migraines are very common. Trigeminal autonomic cephalgias, on the other hand, are much rarer, but the rate of refractoriness to treatment among these patients is significantly higher. Back in 2003, it was suggested that transformed migraine headache may be responsive to occipital PNS [9], and, ever since, the use of PNS in treatment of migraines has attracted the attention of pain practitioners, pain sufferers, and device manufacturers, who have responded by putting together several multicenter prospective randomized clinical trials [10,11,12] one of which led to regulatory approval of occipital PNS for treatment of chronic migraine headaches in Europe in 2011. The autonomic features of migraine headaches and trigeminal autonomic cephalgias brought attention to the sphenopalatine ganglion

(SPG) as a potential target for peripheral neuromodulation [13]. After original encouraging clinical reports, multicenter studies are underway to investigate safety, feasibility, and efficacy of SPG stimulation for various headache and pain indications.

Other less common headache and facial pain disorders, such as hypnic headaches, persistent idiopathic facial pain, post-stroke and multiple sclerosis-associated facial pain have also been treated with either occipital or trigeminal PNS. Moreover, the disabling facial pain syndrome of post-herpetic neuralgia, which frequently involves the ophthalmic branch distribution and usually affects patients of advanced age, has been treated with supraorbital PNS, but its success has been variable.

Lastly, occipital PNS has been successfully used for treatment of pain associated with fibromyalgia [14]. A prospective randomized study is currently underway to investigate the effectiveness of occipital PNS in this condition, which otherwise is not considered a surgical target.

Patient selection criteria

Craniofacial PNS is recommended to a relatively small portion of patients with pain in the craniofacial region. The usual criteria for patient selection are as follows:

(1) The pain has to be chronic: it would not make sense to consider surgical intervention, albeit minimally invasive, to control acute pain that is likely to improve as the tissues heal. The most common criterion for chronicity is pain lasting for 6–12 months, although some centers do not consider the condition chronic if it has lasted less than 3–5 years.

(2) The pain has to be severe: mild or moderate pain syndromes are more responsive to less aggressive approaches, and the risk of surgical intervention may not be justified for less severe pain.

(3) The pain has to be disabling. If it does not affect the patient's quality of life and is simply an unpleasant nuisance, the burden of the procedure in terms of financial and healthcare resource allocation and, most importantly, potential complications, is not justifiable.

(4) The pain has to be refractory to less invasive interventions. This makes sense in terms of risks and complications of PNS. Only when other therapeutic approaches are exhausted, the patient may qualify for PNS. This prerequisite raises potential problems in light of the risks of prolonged medical treatment, particularly opioid therapy, because in the long term, PNS might be safer than potentially harmful and addictive medications. Also, by virtue of being non-destructive, PNS and neuromodulation in general should be considered before any ablative intervention, particularly in those healthcare settings where initial investment in medical device is not cost prohibitive.

(5) The correctable pathology should be corrected whenever possible. It would not make sense to treat occipital neuralgia due to atlanto-occipital instability with PNS when surgical stabilization is likely to eliminate the pain and save the patient from progressive neurological deterioration. Similarly, patients with downward herniation of cerebellar tonsils and the pain was part of the clinical picture of Chiari malformation are more likely to get better from definitive treatment with simple foramen magnum decompression rather than palliative treatment with PNS. At the same time, patients with persistent pain after correction of the underlying pathology are likely to benefit more from pain relieving intervention such as PNS rather than from reoperation.

(6) The diagnosis should be well established and non-responsive conditions should be ruled out. It would not be prudent to consider PNS in patients with craniofacial pain before completion of diagnostic work-up, as sometimes pain may be a presenting symptom of underlying neoplastic, vascular, or inflammatory process. By the same token, some conditions that are known not to respond to electrical stimulation, such as classical trigeminal neuralgia, should not be considered for PNS but instead recommended to have definitive surgery such as microvascular decompression, percutaneous ablation with radiofrequency, glycerol or balloon compression, or stereotactic radiosurgery, each of which may eliminate neuralgic pain permanently or for a long time.

(7) The patient has favorable psychological evaluation. The purpose of psychological evaluation before considering neuromodulation procedures is to assess the chances of response to PNS because patients with dementia, somatization, secondary gain, untreated depression, personality disorder, drug addiction, and other "red flags" are unlikely to benefit from neuromodulation.

(8) The patient does not have a medical condition that would require ongoing magnetic resonance imaging (MRI). This criterion is related to the current state of neuromodulation hardware that is either "MRI-unsafe" or "conditionally safe," meaning that MRI scanning is either completely contraindicated or can be done on very specific parameters. Most likely, this issue will be resolved within the next few years since every device manufacturer is trying to develop MRI-safe equipment.

(9) The patient should not have medical contraindication to the PNS procedure. These include active infection, coagulopathy, inability to stop antiplatelet or anticoagulation treatment, and poor medical condition that would prevent the patient from undergoing sedation or general anesthesia.

(10) Finally, the patient should demonstrate benefit from PNS during the PNS trial. Similar to SCS, the purpose of the trial is to establish effectiveness of the modality, usually defined as more than 50% improvement in pain intensity and the absence of side effects associated with stimulation. There are some exceptions to this rule, for example in some conditions (e.g., cluster headaches) PNS does not produce immediate

improvement and may become effective several weeks or months after device implantation. In these cases, the trial may be helpful in defining whether PNS elicits any undesirable side effects.

Hardware for peripheral nerve stimulation in the craniofacial region

Historically, the devices used in PNS in the head and neck were the same electrode leads, anchors, and generators that were used and approved for use in SCS applications. Despite the fact that the very first electrodes for trigeminal nerve stimulation were custom designed for this application (at that time SCS had not been invented) [15], all subsequent clinical studies and publications have used standard SCS hardware. Even in studies used for regulatory approval of occipital PNS for migraine headaches, the electrodes and implantable pulse generators (IPGs) used were intended for epidural stimulation of the dorsal columns. Most often, the PNS system would include one or several multicontact electrodes that have 4, 8, or 16 contacts each, optional extension cable or cables, and an IPG, either a prime-cell or rechargeable, depending on power requirements, patient, and surgeon preferences, and product availability.

The electrodes traditionally divided into two groups. The cylindrical, wire-like electrodes were designed for insertion through a needle. They are usually called percutaneous electrodes since their insertion does not require extensive surgical exploration and may be done with a percutaneous (as opposed to open) approach. Percutaneous electrodes deliver electrical energy in all directions and this may be preferred for some locations and applications. Other types of electrodes are flat or paddle-like, with electrical contacts facing in one direction and an insulated back-surface that prevents spread of electrical energy toward the back of the lead. These electrodes, sometimes referred to as "laminectomy-type," usually require an open surgical exposure and direct identification of the underlying stimulation target, and in case of PNS—the peripheral nerve. By virtue of their size and shape, paddle electrodes are less likely to migrate, which may be a serious consideration for craniofacial PNS applications. The paddle leads, at least theoretically, may be associated with lower power requirements because of their monodirectional rather than circumferential stimulation. Recently introduced narrow paddle electrodes may be inserted through a wider plastic sheath, combining minimal invasiveness of implantation similar to cylindrical percutaneous leads with lower migration rates and lower power requirements of standard paddle leads.

The electrodes usually require an anchor to be kept in place, and there are multiple models of such anchors ranging from simple silicone tubes with suture holes or grooves for ties to various complex locking devices with metal or hard plastic components. It has to be kept in mind that anchoring the leads too strongly may be associated with higher lead fracture rates, whereas too loose anchoring will not prevent the electrode from migrating. Placing anchors in craniofacial PNS presents a particular challenge as any high-profile system component may create discomfort and its cosmetic appearance may not be acceptable by the patient. Therefore, one must consider the direction of the electrode, choice of anchor, and the location of insertion sites and incisions when treating pain in the head and face of patients.

The power source for craniofacial PNS usually consists of a standard prime cell non-rechargeable IPG (the most common device used for this application worldwide) or a smaller (and usually more versatile) rechargeable IPG. Both of these types of devices provide multiple stimulation options, including range of stimulation frequencies, pulse widths, amplitudes, and cycling options. As technology progressed from externally powered radiofrequency coupled receivers to 4-, 8-, and 16-contact IPGs, so did the choice of stimulation paradigms where multiple combinations of cathodes and anodes allow the electrical field to be shaped in accordance with the individual requirements of each patient.

There are, however, devices that are either specifically designed for craniofacial PNS or developed for other non-SCS applications, with PNS of head and neck being one of them. An example of such development is the BION device [16]. In short, it is a miniaturization in neuromodulation, and the electrode contacts, rechargeable battery, programming and telemetry units can all fit into a single cylindrical stricture smaller than a matchstick that can be "injected" into the living tissue through a small introducer. This device has been successfully tried for treatment of migraines and other headache disorders but still lacks regulatory approval for any pain indications.

Another example of non-SCS devices is a novel stimulator that is specifically designed for stimulation of the SPG [17]. It is intended for implantation in the patient's face using an intraoral approach and is powered by an external hand-held controller that is placed over the receiver part of the implant. The stimulating contacts are inserted into the pterygopalatine fossa in the direct vicinity of the SPG. This stimulation system has now been tested in the treatment of migraines and cluster headaches.

Complications of peripheral nerve stimulation and their avoidance

The surgical procedure to implant a craniofacial PNS device is straightforward. Despite its simplicity, it has several important nuances, each of which is intended to prevent very specific complications.

For the trial phase, the electrode is inserted in the vicinity of the target nerve(s). The choice of the nerve to be stimulated is dictated by the location and pattern of pain; most common targets for stimulation are the greater and lesser occipital nerves, and the supraorbital, infraorbital, and auriculotemporal nerves. It is paramount to avoid injury to the target nerve, and the electrode is implanted at the right depth, between the subcutaneous tissue and the fascia. This epifascial placement appears to be optimal for PNS purposes. Implantation of the stimulating lead under the fascia has been linked to development of stimulation-induced muscle spasms requiring revision of the leads [18]. More superficial placement of the lead may result in lead erosion through the skin, and this complication usually necessitates removal of the lead because the device becomes non-sterile [19].

The lead may be placed either parallel to the target nerve, allowing several electrode contacts to be used for stimulation, or it may be inserted at an angle to the course of the nerve, most often perpendicular to it. This way, the nerve ends up between some of the contacts giving the implanter some freedom in lead positioning and allowing compensation for minor lead migration with simple reprogramming of the device.

Since most nerves in the craniofacial region tend to travel in vertical direction, we prefer placing our PNS electrodes in the horizontal direction, either over the inferior nuchal line for occipital nerve stimulation, just above the eyebrow for the supraorbital nerve stimulation, or a few millimeters below the inferior edge of the orbit for infraorbital nerve stimulation.

To reduce the incidence of infections, we plan the exit site for the trial lead away from the eventual course of the permanent implant. We also keep our patients on oral antibiotics for the duration of the trial with a clear understanding that there is no scientific rationale for such prophylactic use of antibiotic medications.

The use of intraoperative fluoroscopy is recommended for electrode insertion, not for visualization of the target (this may be accomplished with intraoperative ultrasound [20]) but to make sure the lead does not dislodge during tunneling and anchoring.

The implantation of the permanent system in our practice is done under general anesthesia. The pocket for IPG is usually created in the infraclavicular region, and the anchors for the leads are placed in the retroauricular opening. We routinely use manufacturer-recommended anchors in order to minimize complications. As discussed earlier, loose anchoring may result in lead migration, while too tight anchoring (as in direct suturing of the lead to the fascia) may inadvertently damage the inner or outer insulation of the lead resulting in either lead fracture or short circuit, which would necessitate device revision with lead repositioning in case of migration or lead replacement in case of fracture or short circuit.

One way to prevent lead-related complications is to create strain relief loops next to the anchor and the IPG. This maneuver requires somewhat wider dissection at the anchoring site and does not eliminate the need for adequate anchoring of the lead. Needless to say, the anchoring of the IPG and the lead anchor is performed with non-absorbable sutures, and the anchors are attached to the underlying fascial layer. Skin erosion and wound infection over the anchors and generators are avoidable by meticulous closure of the incision and by meticulous hemostasis. We also take time to irrigate the incisions with antibiotic solution and making sure that there are no kinks or sharp bends in the course of the implanted wires.

Common programming parameters

The choice of stimulation parameters greatly depends on the position of the stimulation electrode relative to the nerve to be stimulated. Our usual preference is to use a bipolar set-up with a cathode and anode placed around the stimulated nerve. We almost never use a monopolar set-up (with the IPG case serving as anode) as monopolar stimulation may be uncomfortable for the patient. Sometimes, a simple bipolar set-up is augmented by additional cathodes and anodes either in a "guarded cathode" configuration with positive-negative-positive electrode contact, or as a wider cathode with multiple "positive contacts" next to each other.

The frequency and pulse width are chosen based on the patient's response and perceived pattern of stimulation. We prefer starting patients on the lower pulse width (60-90 μs) and at 40 Hz frequency and then adjust it, usually by increasing both the pulse width and the frequency until the paresthesia coverage is optimal.

The option to control the stimulation amplitude is given to the patient; the clinician's role is to create a range within which the patient can carry out amplitude adjustments. Usually this range corresponds to the so-called "therapeutic window," which starts at the perception threshold (lower limit) and goes up to the discomfort threshold (upper limit). This therapeutic range may have to be adjusted during reprogramming sessions based on the patient's response.

Outcomes and conclusions

In craniofacial pain, PNS appears to be an attractive minimally invasive non-destructive therapeutic option. However, there are several important limitations to its wider acceptance.

There are no standardized, validated diagnostic tests to confirm the diagnosis in most pain syndromes where PNS may be utilized. This refers not only to the diagnostic work-up and terminology, but also to the objective outcome measures.

Another drawback is that there is no dedicated equipment for PNS interventions. Most or all hardware that is used today has been developed, approved, and marketed for SCS applications. Use of inappropriate hardware is at least in part responsible for the very high rate of complications and reoperations. The complication rate in PNS varies from 25% to 100% in long-term follow-up.

There is also no standard surgical technique for PNS, and it varies significantly from one implanting center to another and from one implanter to another. Variations include device location, electrode type and configuration, direction of insertion, position of the generator pocket, choice of anchors, and anchoring technique, all of which are likely to influence short-term and long-term outcome of PNS procedures.

Finally, there is a major shortage of well-designed prospective studies that could validate the value of PNS and document its clinical efficacy and safety. With the exception of several prospective multicenter studies investigating occipital PNS for migraine headaches, most of the published literature (including several recently published books on PNS) is based on retrospective analysis of single-center experiences, and in the era of evidence-based medicine this level of evidence is clearly insufficient.

Despite these limitations, it appears that recent regulatory approval of occipital PNS for refractory migraine headaches is an important step towards establishing the legitimacy of craniofacial PNS. In addition, growing clinical experience with other PNS indications is likely to further refine patient selection criteria and surgical techniques. Moreover, development and clinical introduction of dedicated PNS devices is likely to advance the field toward minimization of complications and improvement in patient outcomes.

Further reading

Abejón, D. & Krames, E.S. (2009) *Peripheral nerve stimulation or is it peripheral subcutaneous field stimulation; what is in a moniker? Neuromodulation*, **12**, 1-4.

Levy, R.M. (2011) *Differentiating the leaves from the branches in the tree of neuromodulation: the state of peripheral nerve field stimulation. Neuromodulation*, **14**, 201-205.

Slavin, K.V. (2008) *Peripheral nerve stimulation for neuropathic pain. Neurotherapeutics*, **5**, 100-106.

Slavin, K.V. (ed.) (2011) *Peripheral Nerve Stimulation*. Karger, Basel.

References

1 Wall, P.D. & Sweet, W.H. (1967) *Temporary abolition of pain in man. Science*, **155**, 108-109.

2 Slavin, K.V. (2011) *History of peripheral nerve stimulation. Progress in Neurological Surgery*, **24**, 1-15.

3 Weiner, R.L. & Reed, K.L. (1999) *Peripheral neurostimulation for control of intractable occipital neuralgia. Neuromodulation*, **2**, 217-221.

4 Picaza, J.A., Hunter, S.E. & Cannon, B.W. (1977-1978) *Pain suppression by peripheral nerve stimulation. Chronic effects of implanted devices. Applied Neurophysiology*, **40**, 223-234.

5 Slavin, K.V., Nersesyan, H. & Wess, C. (2006) *Peripheral neurostimulation for treatment of intractable occipital neuralgia. Neurosurgery*, **58**, 112-119.

6 Slavin, K.V. & Wess, C. (2005) *Trigeminal branch stimulation for intractable neuropathic pain: technical note. Neuromodulation*, **8**, 7-13.

7 Amin, S., Buvanendran, A., Park, K.-S. et al. (2008) *Peripheral nerve stimulator for the treatment of supraorbital neuralgia: a retrospective case series*. Cephalalgia: An International Journal of Headache, **28**, 355-359.

8 Van Buyten, J.P. & Hens, C. (2011) *Chronic stimulation of the Gasserian ganglion in patients with trigeminal neuropathy: a case series*. Journal of Neurosurgical Review, **1** (S1), 73-77.

9 Popeney, C.A. & Aló, K.M. (2003) *Peripheral neurostimulation for the treatment of chronic, disabling transformed migraine*. Headache, **43**, 369-375.

10 Saper, J.R., Dodick, D.W., Silberstein, S.D. et al., ONSTIM Investigators (2011) *Occipital nerve stimulation for the treatment of intractable chronic migraine headache: ONSTIM feasibility study*. Cephalalgia: An International Journal of Headache, **31**, 271-285.

11 Lipton, R.B., Goadsby, P.J., Cady, R.K. et al. (2009) *PRISM study: occipital nerve stimulation for treatment-refractory migraine*. Cephalalgia: An International Journal of Headache, **29** (Suppl. 1), 30.

12 Silberstein, S.D., Dodick, D.W., Saper, J. et al. (2012 Oct 23) *Safety and efficacy of peripheral nerve stimulation of the occipital nerves for the management of chronic migraine: results from a randomized, multicenter, double-blinded, controlled study*. Cephalalgia: An International Journal of Headache, **32**, 1165-1179.

13 Oluigbo, C.O., Makonnen, G., Narouze, S. & Rezai, A.R. (2011) *Sphenopalatine ganglion interventions: technical aspects and application*. Progress in Neurological Surgery, **24**, 171-179.

14 Thimineur, M. & De Ridder, D. (2007) *C2 area neurostimulation: a surgical treatment for fibromyalgia*. Pain Medicine (Malden, Mass.), **8**, 639-646.

15 Shelden, C.H. (1966) Depolarization in the treatment of trigeminal neuralgia. Evaluation of compression and electrical methods; clinical concept of neurophysiological mechanism. In: R.S. Knighton & P.R. Dumke (eds), *Pain*, pp. 373-386. Little, Brown, Boston.

16 Burns, B., Watkins, L. & Goadsby, P.J. (2008) *Treatment of hemicrania continua by occipital nerve stimulation with a Bion device: long-term follow-up of a crossover study*. Lancet Neurology, **7**, 1001-1012.

17 Autonomic Technologies, Inc. (2013) http://www.ati-spg.com/us/en/therapy/ati-system/ [accessed 6 March 2013].

18 Hayek, S.M., Jasper, J.F., Deep, D.R. & Narouze, S.N. (2009) *Occipital neurostimulation-induced muscle spasms: implications for lead placement*. Pain Physician, **12**, 867-876.

19 Trentman, T.L., Dodick, D.W., Zimmerman, R.S. & Birch, B.D. (2008) *Percutaneous occipital stimulator tip erosion: report of 2 cases*. Pain Physician, **11**, 253-256.

20 Skaribas, I. & Aló, K. (2010) *Ultrasound imaging and occipital nerve stimulation*. Neuromodulation, **13**, 126-130.

Chapter 23

Peripheral Nerve Stimulation in Pain of the Body and Extremities

Konstantin V. Slavin[1], Sami Al-Nafi[1], and Serge Y. Rasskazoff[2]

[1]University of Illinois at Chicago, Chicago, Illinois, USA
[2]Flint, Michigan, USA

Introduction

In the field of neuromodulation, peripheral nerve stimulation (PNS) has a very special place; despite many decades of clinical use, it is still struggling to become widely used modality along with deep brain stimulation (DBS) and spinal cord stimulation (SCS). This chapter summarizes the current state of PNS in treatment of chronic pain in the body and extremities.

First reports of PNS for the treatment of neuropathic pain were published in the late 1960s. In fact, the famous 1969 book *Pain and the Neurosurgeon* by White and Sweet [1] had a description and an X-ray image of a PNS device implanted on the ulnar nerve of the patient with post-traumatic neuropathy. Since then, dozens of clinical reports have dealt with various aspects of PNS in the 1970s, 1980s, and 1990s, and the procedure of PNS has remained relatively unchanged: the target nerve was exposed and the paddle-type lead was placed in direct contact with the nerve trunk [2]. To facilitate this procedure, a specially designed paddle lead was created; it had an integrated mesh attached to the paddle allowing the surgeon to wrap the lead around the nerve rather than suture it *in situ*.

The introduction of percutaneous PNS insertion techniques in the late 1990s has revolutionized the PNS field [3]. Although this approach appeared to be most applicable to PNS in the craniofacial region, it gradually spread

Neurostimulation: Principles and Practice, First Edition. Edited by Sam Eljamel and Konstantin V. Slavin.
© 2013 John Wiley & Sons, Ltd. Published 2013 by John Wiley & Sons, Ltd.

to PNS in the lower parts of the body, including the extremities, abdomen, chest wall, upper and lower back, groin area, and neck. The next development was the introduction of the peripheral nerve field stimulation (PNFS) concept (sometimes called subcutaneous nerve stimulation, subcutaneous target stimulation, or peripheral field stimulation), which is considered a variation of PNS as it targets more distal neural structures, the unnamed nerve branches, and subcutaneous nerve endings [4]. More recently, the PNS approach was augmented by the addition of ultrasound guidance, which helps in the visualization of peripheral nerves during percutaneous lead insertion [5]. Finally, the progress in PNS is facilitated by several new companies, each of which came up with innovative devices and surgical techniques specifically developed for PNS applications.

Indications and patient selection

The general rules of neuromodulation apply to patient selection in PNS as well. This modality is considered in cases of neuropathic pain that satisfies the general criteria of being chronic, severe, disabling, refractory to medical treatments, associated with clear a diagnostic impression, and occurring in the absence of correctable underlying pathology. In addition, patients are expected to be familiar with the modality and willing to use it, have a favorable neuropsychological profile, and have positively responded to a trial of PNS before the permanent device is implanted. The usual contraindications, such as short life expectancy, active infection, uncorrectable coagulopathy or thrombocytopenia, and generally poor medical condition that would prevent patients from elective surgery and/or anesthesia should all be taken into consideration.

Most common indications for PNS in the extremities are chronic pain due to peripheral nerve injury, persistent pain from compressive neuropathy (following adequate decompression), complex regional pain syndromes (CRPS) type 1 (formerly known as reflex sympathetic dystrophy) and type 2 (formerly known as causalgia), and painful peripheral neuropathy. For PNS (of PNFS) in the chest wall, abdomen, neck, upper and lower back, groin area, and other parts of the trunk, the most common indications are post-surgical neuropathic pain, post-infectious (particularly post-herpetic) pain, and post-traumatic neuropathy. It appears from the literature and personal communication with neuromodulation practitioners worldwide that in the category of PNS below the head and face the previously dominant indications of pain due to peripheral nerve injury and CRPS are now eclipsed by a large number of patients with pain due to failed back surgery syndrome (FBSS). This mainly reflects the much higher prevalence of back pain in the population and is likely to be related to the recent growth in the number of spinal interventions and the general ineffectiveness of other treatment modalities, including SCS, in the management of axial back pain or paraspinal lumbar pain.

It appears that pain in the extremities patients with pain limited to the distribution of a single nerve are better candidates for PNS, whereas pain in the trunk, chest, or abdomen patients with a smaller area of pain may respond better to PNS/PNFS. Also, pure sensory nerves tend to be better targets for PNS than mixed nerves, and PNS delivered to mixed or predominantly motor nerves may be limited due to undesired motor side effects. Another indication for PNS is pain from amputation neuromas, as it might be easier to stimulate the nerve that has become a source of pain and discomfort without serving any useful function.

Device choice

Traditionally, PNS for treatment of pain has been performed with neuromodulation hardware that was intended for SCS. The wrap-around design of the initial custom-made electrode leads has been subsequently used in PNS of phrenic and vagal nerves (for diaphragmal palsy and for epilepsy and depression, respectively). The subsequently developed "multibutton" electrode design was introduced for PNS application, but did not go into mass production. The purpose here was to specifically stimulate separate fascicles of a large mixed nerve, such as the sciatic nerve, but, for a variety of reasons, the standard paddle electrodes that were already available for SCS applications became the preferred PNS delivery device. To overcome the formation of scar tissue between the nerve and the paddle lead, the paddles were modified by attaching an integrated Dacron mesh that could be wrapped around the nerve [6]. However, the open surgical approach with nerve exploration that is required for implantation of paddle leads has become almost completely abandoned with the introduction of percutaneous PNS techniques. However, even now several large-volume practices continue using paddle leads for PNS; this preference is related to several important benefits of the paddle leads. First, modern paddles have several rows of contacts (between one and five rows) that are separated by a pre-set distance. This allows multiple stimulation paradigms to be created in the longitudinal, transverse, and oblique directions with electrode contact configuration that matches the course of sensory fibers inside the nerve trunk. Second, the paddle structure ensures unidirectional stimulation, so electrical energy gets directed toward the nerve while the surrounding tissues are shielded by the paddle lead insulation. A corollary to this, paddle leads are expected to consume less energy to produce the desired effect and, therefore, may be associated with longer life of implantable pulse generators (IPGs). Lastly, the use of paddles in PNS, similar to the SCS experience, is associated with much lower migration rates.

However, the invasiveness of paddle insertion and the need for highly refined surgical skills to expose the peripheral nerves were not the only reasons for the lack of widespread acceptance of paddle-based PNS. Multiple reports of perineural fibrosis following long-term PNS with paddle leads raised concern about their safety and appropriateness. However, this phenomenon occurred in a very small percentage of patients. Nevertheless, percutaneous lead insertion for PNS/PNFS application has become more widespread, and, by some estimates, between 25% and 50% of devices implanted in the USA in 2011 were used for this purpose. Nowadays, percutaneous electrode leads are chosen when the stimulated nerve is located in a predictable area, when stimulation may be delivered without direct contact with the nerve—with the electrode lead aimed parallel to the nerve, perpendicular to it, or in an oblique direction—and whenever the painful area is covered with one or several leads so the paresthesias elicited by these leads are concordant with the pain distribution. In addition, insertion of percutaneous PNS leads may be facilitated by the use of ultrasound guidance, which helps in finding the nerve path and its depth and in avoiding the adjacent vascular structures.

The choice of power source for PNS is usually determined by stimulation energy consumption. In the past (and even now in the USA), the only approved devices for PNS applications were radiofrequency (RF)-coupled systems. In such systems the power source is external; it delivers energy by means of a RF link between the transmitting antenna and an implanted receiver that is connected to the electrodes either directly or via extensions. Once popular because of its relative versatility compared with the first generation of IPGs, RF-coupled systems are rarely if ever used these days. In fact, the new generation of neuromodulation practitioners have probably never seen such device. A prime cell battery powers several models of IPGs, and this meant that the entire device had to be replaced when the battery became depleted. Such depletion could occur within a year after implantation if high-power settings were used during stimulation and if the patient was using stimulation around the clock. The need for frequent IPG replacements was eliminated by the introduction of rechargeable technology. Today, rechargeable IPGs dominate the neuromodulation market, but in some parts of the world this technology is not available because of the lack of regulatory approval or, more often, due to prohibitively high, unaffordable costs. In PNS applications, the use of rechargeable technology makes even more sense than, for example, in DBS or SCS applications: the low profile and smaller size of rechargeable IPGs provide less discomfort and more appealing cosmetic appearance for PNS/PNFS patients.

Interestingly, the old concepts of wrap-around electrode leads and RF-coupled power sources have recently been reborn for PNS applications. Two different start-up companies have placed their main focus on PNS-oriented devices. One company uses specially designed coil-like electrodes to wrap around peripheral nerves while delivering high-frequency electrical stimulation in order to eliminate the pain of amputation neuroma [7]. Another company has developed an RF-coupled implantable system where the electrode itself serves as an antenna linked to an external miniature power source that is taped to the skin over it [8].

Procedural details

The technique of PNS implantation depends on the stimulation target and on the choice of hardware. When plans are for direct stimulation of a specific peripheral nerve, the electrode may be implanted either through open exploration of the nerve segment or with a percutaneous approach in the vicinity of the nerve. In both scenarios, the anatomical knowledge of the nerve course is important, and in the latter one the guidance for electrode insertion may be facilitated with fluoroscopy (to define known skeletal landmarks) or ultrasound (to directly visualize the nerve and adjacent vascular bundle). It is also very important to identify the segment of the stimulated nerve where it is surgically accessible and where nerve branching is minimal. It is even more important to plan the lead position and trajectory from its entry point to its intended final position and tunneling path in such a way that major joints are avoided, for repetitive movements of the lead or extension cable may result in material fatigue and eventual lead fracture. Both metal wires and external plastic insulation may become damaged from constant bending and unbending of the device. Needless to say, surgical expertise in dealing with peripheral nerves is needed for anyone who decides to implant paddle leads for PNS, and great familiarity with intraoperative ultrasound is needed before using it for PNS targeting.

For PNFS applications, on the other hand, detailed knowledge of peripheral nerve anatomy is less essential because the leads are implanted either in the middle of the painful area or at its edges. Traditionally, it has been suggested that a painful area the size of a business card (or a credit card) might be covered with a single cylindrical electrode lead inserted right in its middle. Everything bigger than a credit card—but still within a 10- to 12-cm limit—has to be treated with two leads located on the periphery of the painful region. This conceptual notion was changed with the introduction of the so-called "cross-talk" approach, which postulates an ability to cover very large areas of the body with separate electrode leads placed far from each other [9]. This approach has been validated with some theoretical modeling and in small clinical series but so far has not received widespread acceptance.

One of the practical aspects of lead insertion is electrode depth. It appears that for PNS and PNFS applications, the best depth of the lead is just above the deep subcutaneous fascia. Placing leads in the epifascial plane eliminates muscle spasms that occur when the lead is placed too deep, and minimizes the risk of lead erosion which may happen if the lead is placed too superficially. The depth should also be considered when choosing an appropriate anchoring device, as some of the commercially available anchors have too big a profile that may produce discomfort or visibly deform the skin, or, in some cases, end up eroding through the skin. Nevertheless, anchoring electrode lead(s) in place is an important step in device implantation since the high mobility of soft tissues in PNS/PNFS applications may result in an even higher migration rate than keeping them in a relatively immobile epidural space in SCS or using skull-mounted fixation of leads in DBS. Whatever the anchor or the anchoring technique used for PNS devices, the general recommendation is to use non-absorbable sutures and fix the lead to a hard tissue, such as thick deep fascia. In addition to anchoring, it is recommended to use so-called "strain relief" loops, which are intended to minimize lead displacement during the patient's body movement. These loops should be placed, if possible, next to the anchor (between the anchor and the generator) and next to the IPG. This approach should further minimize electrode migration or fracture.

Finally, the location and depth of IPG implantation have to be well thought of and pre-planned. The position of the IPG in PNS is usually dictated by the location of pain and, subsequently, the stimulating electrode leads. Placing the IPG over bony prominences (edge of the rib cage, iliac crest, scapula) or too close to the midline should be avoided to prevent patient discomfort. Burying the IPG deep into the soft tissues may interfere with the ability to recharge the device, but putting it immediately under the dermis increases the risk of poor wound healing, device erosion, and implant site pain.

Evidence base

The long-term outcome of more recently introduced PNFS is still unknown. Large series from Australia and Europe, some of which were used for gaining regulatory approval on these continents, discussed outcomes at 3 months in a heterogeneous cohort of 111 patients (the Austrian multicenter study [10]) and 7 months in 13 patients (the Australian experience [11]). All published studies documented, consistently observed more than a 50% reduction in the pain level in every group of PNS/PNFS patients.

In traditional PNS cases, much longer follow up has been summarized in multiple publications. An average follow-up of more than 10 years in a combined German–Israeli experience of Dr. Waisbrod showed that among 46 implanted PNS patients, good results were observed in 22 out of 30 (73%) of the lower extremity implants and in 10 out of 12 (83%) of the upper extremity implants [12]. The patients with post-surgical nerve injury and entrapment neuropathy exhibited significant improvement in more than 80% of cases, while those with pain after traumatic injections had a 50% success rate, and those with pain after nerve graft–0%. Even longer follow-up (more than 20 years) was reported in the Belgian study of Drs. Van Calenbergh and Gybels where patients implanted in the 1980s continued to enjoy more than 50% improvement in pain intensity when using their PNS devices [13].

Common programming parameters

There are no hard rules on PNS/PNFS parameters and programming. The goal of stimulation is to cover the painful region with paresthesias and avoid unpleasant sensations from stimulation. The polarity of the electrode contacts varies from a simple bipolar set-up when the cathode and anode are next to each other to somewhat more complex paradigms where the cathode and anode are placed at opposite ends of the electrode lead, or the lead configuration involves multiple cathodes and anodes in continuous (−−−−++++) or intermittent (+−+−+−+−) fashion. The cross-talk paradigm mentioned earlier also explored placing cathodes on one lead and the anodes on the other, thereby spreading the electrical field.

Other parameters of stimulation (pulse width, frequency and amplitude) are also individually tailored. Most commonly, the pulse width is between 90 μs and 300 μs, and the frequency is between 20 Hz and 80 Hz. Lower frequency is sometimes perceived by the patient as an unpleasant thumping, whereas higher frequency may be felt as painful. The amplitude is individually adjusted between onset of perception and development of stimulation-induced discomfort. In "constant voltage" devices (e.g., Medtronic), the amplitude is usually between 2 and 6 V, and in "constant current" devices (e.g., St. Jude Medical and Boston Scientific), the amplitude is between 1 and 7 mAmp.

Similar to other neuromodulation applications, the patient gets an option of changing stimulation parameters (usually only the amplitude, but sometimes also frequency and pulse width) using his/her "patient controller" within a pre-set range that is established by the programming team (physician, nurse, or medical assistant, and the representative of device manufacturer) using a "physician programmer." Very frequently, the patient also has an option to switch between different programs that are set to be more useful for various body positions, activity levels, or pain fluctuations.

Conclusions

The peripheral neuromodulation approach includes the following three modalities: (1) PNS, which requires implantation of stimulating electrode leads over the affected peripheral nerves, (2) percutaneous PNS, which involves insertion of leads in the vicinity of the nerve with proper guidance, and (3) PNFS, which stimulates smaller nerves and nerve endings in the region of pain. It is an effective way to control chronic, disabling, medically refractory neuropathic pain of different etiologies. PNS is expected to become accepted (and properly covered by the regulatory agencies and payers) once more prospective evidence of its long-term clinical efficacy and cost-effectiveness becomes available.

The introduction of dedicated PNS/PNFS devices is needed to reduce complication rates and improve reliability in obtaining optimal outcomes. Based on our observations and expectations, the next decade will bring both technical advances and clinical experience in the PNS/PNFS arena.

References

1 White, J.C. & Sweet, W.H. (1969) *Pain and the Neurosurgeon. A Forty-Year Experience*, p. 894. Thomas, Springfield, IL.

2 Slavin, K.V. (2011) History of peripheral nerve stimulation. *Progress in Neurological Surgery*, **24**, 1–15.

3 Weiner, R.L. & Reed, K.L. (1999) Peripheral neurostimulation for control of intractable occipital neuralgia. *Neuromodulation*, **2**, 217–221.

4 Abejon, D. & Perez-Cajaraville, J. (2011) Peripheral nerve stimulation: definition. *Progress in Neurological Surgery*, **24**, 203–209.

5 Huntoon, M.A. & Burgher, A.H. (2009) Ultrasound-guided permanent implantation of peripheral nerve stimulation (PNS) system for neuropathic pain of the extremities: original cases and outcomes. *Pain Medicine (Malden, Mass.)*, **10**, 1369–1377.

6 Mobbs, R.J., Blum, P. & Rossato, R. (2003) Mesh electrode for peripheral nerve stimulation. *Journal of Clinical Neuroscience*, **10**, 476–477.

7 Soin, A., Kilgore, K., Bhadra, N. & Fang, Z.P. (2011) Feasibility study on high-frequency electrical nerve block for amputation pain. *Neuromodulation*, **14**, 561.

8 Deer, T.R., Levy, R.M. & Rosenfeld, E.L. (2010) Prospective clinical study of a new implantable peripheral nerve stimulation device to treat chronic pain. *The Clinical Journal of Pain*, **26**, 359–372.

9 Falco, F.J.E., Berger, J., Vrable, A. *et al.* (2009) Cross talk: a new method for peripheral nerve stimulation. An observational report with cadaveric verification. *Pain Physician*, **12**, 965–983.

10 Sator-Katzenschlager, S., Fiala, K., Kress, H.G. *et al.* (2010) Subcutaneous target stimulation (STS) in chronic noncancer pain: a nationwide retrospective study. *Pain Practice*, **10**, 279–286.

11 Verrills, P., Mitchell, B., Vivian, D. & Sinclair, C. (2009) Peripheral nerve stimulation: a treatment for chronic low back pain and failed back surgery syndrome? *Neuromodulation*, **12**, 68–75.

12 Eisenberg, E., Waisbrod, H. & Gerbershagen, H.U. (2004) Long-term peripheral nerve stimulation for painful nerve injuries. *The Clinical Journal of Pain*, **20**, 143–146.

13 Van Calenbergh, F., Gybels, J., Van Laere, K. *et al.* (2009) Long term clinical outcome of peripheral nerve stimulation in patients with chronic peripheral neuropathic pain. *Surgical Neurology*, **72**, 330–335.

Appendix I

Principles of Programming of Neurostimulators

Sam Eljamel, Patrick Carena, and Catherine Young

Ninewells Hospital and Medical School, Dundee, UK

Although patient and target selection, and precise and accurate implantation of the neurostimulator play the most important roles to achieve the goals of neurostimulation therapy, programming the neurostimulator is as important. The possible combinations of programming parameters is more than the possible combinations of the national lottery, and you will not be wrong to conclude it would be impossible to go through all the possible combinations, making finding the right winning combination as elusive as winning the lottery. Despite what seems to be an impossible task or mission impossible, in reality programming can be very quick and easy to find the right programming parameters for a particular patient because the programmer is guided by the following foresights:

(1) Choosing the most effective contact out of possible four is often guided by post-implantation neuroimaging (Figures AI.1 and AI.2).
(2) Previous reported experience, e.g., most patients will respond well to a rate of 130 Hz.
(3) Responses to intraoperative stimulation or trial stimulation.

In our institution we found the following guidance very useful in finding out the best programming parameters for a particular patient:

(1) Measure the impedance of both leads at the end of implanting the IPG to make sure that all circuits are properly connected. The impedance should be <2000 ohms. If the impedance was >2000 ohms or high there must be a break in the circuit, which needs to be resolved prior to programming.

Neurostimulation: Principles and Practice, First Edition. Edited by Sam Eljamel and Konstantin V. Slavin.
© 2013 John Wiley & Sons, Ltd. Published 2013 by John Wiley & Sons, Ltd.

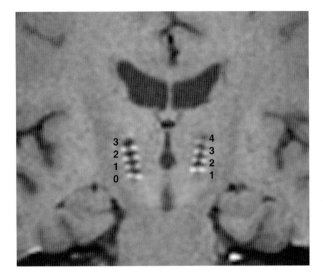

Figure AI.1 Coronal magnetic resonance image demonstrating the position of deep brain stimulation leads-contacts in relation to the STN (right contacts numbered 0–3 for Medtronic lead and left contacts numbered 1–4 for St. Jude Medical lead).

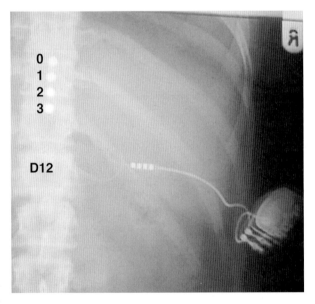

Figure AI.2 Anteroposterior radiograph demonstrating the position of Resume lead in spinal cord stimulation.

(2) Wait for the acute effects of lead implantation to settle prior to starting programming. The reason for this wait is to allow the impedance to return to normal as the impedance in the first week or so might be artificially low because of acute surgical effects and trauma. In our institution we wait for 2 weeks before beginning programming. Another

reason for this wait is to allow any postoperative edema, pain or swelling at the IPG site to settle.

(3) Program the IPG case as positive (anode), the pulse width at 60 to 90 µs and a rate of 130 Hz.

(4) Program the most distal contact as negative (cathode) (this would be contact 0 or 5 in the Medtronic dual channel device and 1 in St. Jude Medical device.

(5) Increase the amplitude gradually and slowly from 0 to the maximum tolerated amplitude:

  (a) Observe any side effects:

    (i) Sensory side effects, e.g., tingling and paresthesia and record its location, e.g., the face, the tongue, the hand, or leg.

    (ii) Motor side effects, e.g., pulling or twitching of the face, arm, or leg. Please record its location as above.

    (iii) Any other side effects, e.g., speech disturbance or speech arrest, dizziness, headache, diplopia, giddiness, or imbalance.

  (b) Observe the effects of stimulation on the symptoms, e.g., tremor suppression, dyskinesia suppression, or reduction of rigidity.

  (c) The amplitude range that provides relief of symptoms without major side effects is called the therapeutic window, e.g., if an amplitude of 2 provides benefit and intolerable side effects occur at 5, then the therapeutic window is 2-4.9.

(6) Find the therapeutic window for each contact as per the previous step and record beneficial response and potential side effects.

(7) Compare the best response at each therapeutic window.

(8) Use the contact that provided the best therapy as your primary program in monopolar setting.

(9) Adjust the pulse width, rate, and amplitude to maximize the benefits of stimulation.

(10) You might also use more than one contact if necessary or bipolar if that program produced better results.

(11) It is very important however to have the initial therapeutic window of each contact or combination of contacts in front of you in any future programming sessions to avoid exceeding the threshold of safe stimulation as exceeding the threshold of safe stimulation is likely to alarm the patient, remind him/her of the initial session and it may also exacerbate the symptoms, e.g., tremor. Exacerbation of symptoms during programming often prolongs the programming session.

(12) It is also paramount that you record the programming parameters in the patient's records or the patient's card.

(13) It is also important to check the impedance before altering programming to ensure that the electric circuits are intact. High impedance or an impedance above 2000 ohms indicates that a break in the system (please check Appendix 2 for trouble shooting malfunctioning neurostimulator system).

Appendix II

Troubleshooting Malfunctioning Neurostimulators

Sam Eljamel

Centre for Neurosciences, University of Dundee, Ninewells Hospital and Medical School, Dundee, UK

The response and proper function of any neurostimulator system is dependent on the following factors:

(1) Selection of the right patient.
(2) Tailoring the right target to the right patient.
(3) Tailoring programming to each patient.
(4) Continuing follow up and patient education.

However, anyone involved in implanting neurostimulation systems and follow-up of patients with implanted systems will know well that despite adhering to the above four pillars of successful neurostimulation programs, neurostimulation systems will often develop a problem that needs fixing. The following guide will cover most of the encountered problems and provides some of the possible solutions.

Loss of response

The most common cause of lack of response is a hardware problem:

(1) depleted battery
(2) break in the electric circuit
(3) lead migration.

Neurostimulation: Principles and Practice, First Edition. Edited by Sam Eljamel and Konstantin V. Slavin.
© 2013 John Wiley & Sons, Ltd. Published 2013 by John Wiley & Sons, Ltd.

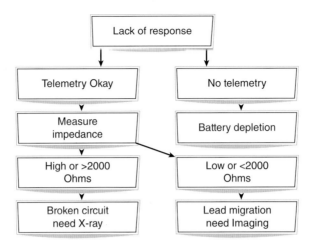

Figure AII.1 Flow chart to diagnose and resolve lack of neurostimulator response.

Figure AII.1 demonstrates a flow chart revealing the underlying cause of lost response of neurostimulator systems.

First interrogate the IPG to assess the battery charge. If you cannot communicate with the IPG the battery is most likely to have been depleted. If you can communicate with the IPG, measure the impedance. If the impedance was high or >2000 ohms, the system must have developed an electric break somewhere along the system from the IPG header to the contacts.

Battery depletion

Battery depletion comes to attention when patients are unable to communicate with the IPG or patients report loss of response. Loss of response can be confirmed by inability of the physician programmer to communicate with or interrogate the IPG. An error message, "cannot communicate or can not find the IPG, please position the wand on the IPG and try again," will be displayed on the physician programmer's screen.

A depleted battery can be resolved by replacing the IPG with an identical IPG or a newer model. Newer models may require an adaptor (please consult the manufacturer regarding compatibility). In some patients, e.g., those who require high-amplitude stimulation that drains the battery quickly, it might be better to replace the IPG by a rechargeable battery if the patient is able and willing to use such rechargeable battery to avoid loss of response of the system when the battery is depleted.

High impedance

High impedance indicates a broken electric circuit. Broken circuit may occur due to loosening of the IPG lead extender connections or more commonly

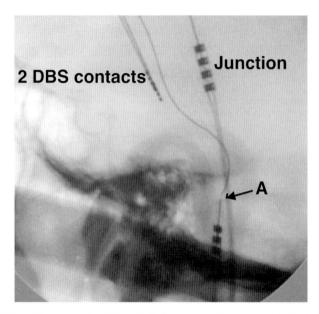

Figure AII.2 Radiograph of the skull demonstrating a break in the lead about 10 mm proximal to the lead-lead extender junction (A). DBS, deep brain stimulation.

following lead fractures. Lead fractures occur in 0–13%. The most common site of lead fractures in DBS is about 10 mm proximal to lead-lead extender junction (Figure AII.2) and at the exit of the deep spinal fascia in SCS. Plain radiographs of the whole system may identify the exact location of the break, but sometimes the break is not visible on X-rays because it is microscopic in nature.

To avoid DBS lead fractures, position the lead-lead extender junction in the parietal region and use long enough lead extender to permit leaving lead extender loop behind the IPG or in the neck to provide slack for neck movements. Alternatively use flexible stretchable lead extenders.

In SCS leave a loop of the lead deeper to the deep fascia of the spine, distal to the anchor. Sometimes high impedance in SCS is due to epidural fibrosis rather than hardware failure. Broken leads need to be replaced. During replacement the continuity of the electric circuit can be tested and the leads can be inspected under the microscope [1].

Low impedance

Loss of stimulation system beneficial response associated with low or <2000 ohms impedance most likely is due to lead migration or imprecise position or inadequate fixation of the lead (Figure AII.3).

Lead migration used to occur in about 14%. However, with the advent of new technology and evolution of the surgical technique, lead migration had

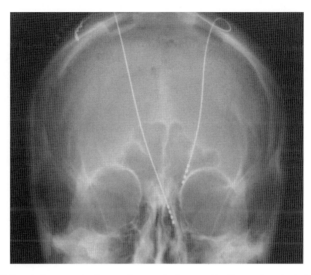

Figure AII.3 Anteroposterior radiograph demonstrating migrated right deep brain stimulation lead.

been reduced to merely 0-5%. Lead migration can be avoided by adequate lead fixation using the manufacturer's lead fixation anchors to fix the DBS lead to the skull or to fix the SCS lead to the spinal fascia. Some surgeons use miniplates to fix the DBS lead to the skull. It is important to avoid crushing the DBS lead if miniplate and screws are used. To avoid electrical failure in these circumstances it would be advisable to protect the DBS lead by small piece of silicone or plastic.

Low impedance <250 ohms often is due to short circuit along the system. This can be caused by a breakdown of the insulation and patients may feel unpleasant tingling sensation in the area where the electric leak is located.

Narrow therapeutic window

The most common cause of narrow therapeutic window is imperfect positioning of the stimulator lead or lead migration. For this reason most centers perform postoperative imaging to confirm the exact positions of the four contacts in relation to the intended target. In SCS, plain radiographs in the anteroposterior and lateral planes will be sufficient to confirm the epidural location of the SCS and at what spinal level and its laterality (Figure AII.2 and Figure AII.4).

In DBS there are two ways of confirming the final position of the contacts:

(1) MRI (Figure AI.1): If the MRI safety protocol at your institution permits performing MRI scans in patients with implanted neurostimulator systems, follow exactly what the manufacturer of the system recommends. The

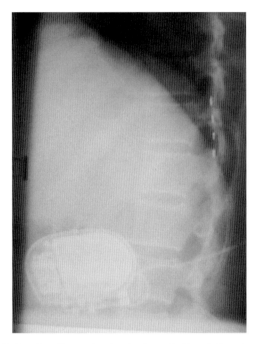

Figure AII.4 Lateral radiograph of spinal cord stimulation demonstrating the epidural position.

main concerns of performing MRI in patients with DBS in place are damage to the neurostimulator system itself, nerve tissue damage due heating of the DBS system, and ferromagnetic artifacts degrading the diagnostic quality of the MRI. MRI is contraindicated in patients with neurostimulator using full body transmit radiofrequency coil, receive only head coil or head transmit coil that extends over the chest. Performing MRI with these types of coils heats the DBS and can cause paralysis, coma, or even death. Medtronic, for example, recommends the following procedure:

a. The MRI must be absolutely necessary and the desired diagnostic information could not be obtained in any other safer way, e.g., using CT.

b. An MRI radiologist or physicist is satisfied that all safety procedures are followed.

c. Patient was informed of the risk of MRI with DBS *in situ*.

d. MRI performed awake so the patient can give feedback.

e. Any exteriorized leads or lead extenders must be insulated and positioned straight in the center of the coil without a loop.

f. Make sure that no open circuit exists by measuring the impedance. If the circuit was open do not perform an MRI scan.

g. MRI should not be performed on a broken or fractured lead.

   h. Neurostimulator setting must be:
      i.   Output should be off.
      ii. Amplitude set to zero.
      iii. Stimulation mode should be bipolar.
      iv. Cycling should be disabled.
      v.   Magnetic stimulation should be disabled.
   i. MRI settings must be:
      i.   Use only horizontal tube 1.5 Tesla MRI machine.
      ii. Use only transmit/receive head coil that does not extend over the chest or neck.
      iii. Enter the exact weight of the patient in the MRI machine software.
      iv. Use MRI parameters that limit the SAR to 0.1 W/kg.
      v.   Limit the gradient dB/dt field to 20 tesla/s or less.
(2) CT (Figure AII.5): CT that can be merged with the planning MR image can provide adequate localization of the DBS contacts in almost all patients. This is a much safer option.

Skin erosions and infections

A number of patients with implanted neurostimulators will develop skin erosion around the neurostimulator system e.g. around the IPG (Figure AII.6), around the lead-lead extender or the burr hole cap.

The best strategy to avoid skin erosion is prevention. The following techniques have been used to minimize skin erosions.

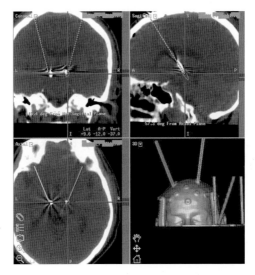

Figure AII.5 Screenshot of fused post DBS implantation CT merged with the preoperative MRI-based targets demonstrating perfect alignment of the plan trajectories and target to the implanted DBS leads. Refer to color plate section for color version of this figure.

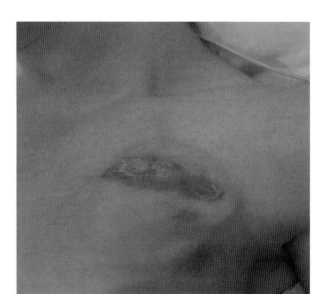

Figure AII.6 Skin erosion over the implantable pulse generator in a patient with dystonia.

(1) Using curved incisions over the DBS entry point. This may also reduce the incidence of infection.
(2) Drilling a small trench in the outer table of the skull to receive the lead-lead extender junction or using low profile connecter.
(3) Making sure the skin over the IPG is of good quality or burying the IPG under the pectoralis muscle. Using smaller IPG can also help.

Skin erosion can often be treated by repositioning the IPG or the component and provide a good skin coverage (Figure AII.7).

However, more often than not skin erosions are associated with chronic or acute infection. Infections can occur in 2–15% of neurostimulation procedures. Staged procedures where the leads are exteriorized for a period of time are associated with higher risk of infection than those, which were performed without exteriorization (in DBS 15.3% versus 4.2% [2]). When skin incisions cross directly over the neurostimulator hardware the risk of infection is also much higher than when the hardware does not cross skin incisions (e.g., in DBS infection when straight incision was performed across the burr hole was 12% compared to 2% when small skin flap was performed to cover the burr hole [2]). It is possible to avoid the hardware crossing skin incisions as follows:

(1) In the scalp make small curved flap over the entry burr hole with the base of the flap where you intend the lead to go posterior.
(2) Over the lead-lead extender junction you can make the incision posterior where to intend to position the junctions.

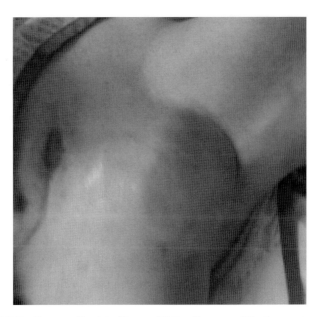

Figure AII.7 Same patient in Figure AII.6, after repositioning.

Table AII.1 Summary of successful intravenous antibiotic therapy in infected neurostimulation systems

Authors	Number of infected systems	Successful antibiotic therapy alone (%)
Oh *et al.* [3]	6	1 (17)
Kumar *et al.* [4]	4	3 (75)
DBS study group [5]	4	2 (50)
Levy *et al.* [6]	23	1 (4)
Koller *et al.* [7]	2	2 (100)
Constantoyannis *et al.* [2]	9	3 (33)
Pooled data	48	12 (25)

(3) Behind the auricle make the incision posterior to where the DBS lead extenders will eventually travel.

(4) In the infraclavicular fossa and where the IPG will be located you can make the incision at the bottom of the IPG pocket. This will prevent the IPG from migrating downwards when the surgical scar heals below the IPG and it will also make IPG replacements easier because there are no wires crossing the surgical scar.

If the infection is localized, a trial of intravenous antibiotics might succeed in an average of one out of four patients (Table AII.1). If the infection is major and localized to the IPG site, treat with intravenous antibiotics and remove the IPG. Reimplant a new IPG when the infection is settled completely. If the infection is in or spread to the scalp, the quickest and surest way of getting rid of the infection is to remove the whole system and treat with IV antibiotics before reimplantation of new system.

References

1 Akmal, S. & Eljamel, M.S. (2008) Spinal cord stimulation for chronic pain: causes of long-term paddle-lead failure. *Neuromodulation* **11**, 282-285.

2 Constantoyannis, C., Berk, C., Honey, C.R. *et al.* (2005) Reducing hardware-related complications of deep brain stimulation. *Canadian Journal of Neurological Science* **32**, 194-200.

3 Oh, M.Y., Abosch, A., Kim, S.H. *et al.* (2002) Long term hardware-related complications of deep brain stimulation. *Neurosurgery* **50**, 1268-1276.

4 Kumar, K., Toth, C. & Nath, R. (1997) Deep brain stimulation for intractable pain: a 15-year experience. *Neurosurgery* **40**, 736-747.

5 The Deep Brain Stimulation for Parkinson's Disease Study Group. (2001) Deep brain stimulation of the subthalamic nucleus or the pars interna of the globus pallidus in Parkinson's disease. *New England Journal of Medicine* **345**, 956-963.

6 Levy, R., Lamb, S. & Adams, J. (1987) Treatment of chronic pain by deep brain stimulation: long term follow up and review of the literature. *Neurosurgery* **21**, 885-893.

7 Koller, W., Pawha, R., Busenbark, K. *et al.* (1997) High-frequency unilateral thalamic stimulation in the treatment of essential and parkinsonian tremor. *Annals of Neurology* **42**, 292-299.

Index

Neurostimulation: Principles and Practice, First Edition. Edited by Sam Eljamel and
Konstantin V. Slavin.
© 2013 John Wiley & Sons, Ltd. Published 2013 by John Wiley & Sons, Ltd.